Mastering the UKCAT

Mastering the UKCAT

Dr Christopher Nordstrom
George Rendel
Dr Ricardo Tavares

CRC Press
Taylor & Francis Group
6000 Broken Sound Parkway NW, Suite 300
Boca Raton, FL 33487-2742

Printed on acid-free paper
Version Date: 20150416

International Standard Book Number-13: 978-1-4822-5966-7 (Paperback)

Library of Congress Cataloging-in-Publication Data

Nordstrom, Christopher, author.
   Mastering the UKCAT / Christopher Nordstrom, George Rendel, Ricardo Tavares.
   p. ; cm.
   Mastering the United Kingdom Clinical Aptitude Test
   Includes bibliographical references and index.
   ISBN 978-1-4822-5966-7 (paperback : alk. paper)
   I. Tavares, Ricardo, 1984- , author. II. Rendel, George, 1983- , author. III. Title. IV. Title: Mastering the United Kingdom Clinical Aptitude Test.
   [DNLM: 1. Medicine--Great Britain--Examination Questions. 2. College Admission Test--Great Britain--Examination Questions. W 18.2]

   R838.5
   610.76--dc23
                                                                        2015013885

Visit the Taylor & Francis Web site at
http://www.taylorandfrancis.com

and the CRC Press Web site at
http://www.crcpress.com

Contents

About the Authors

Dr Christopher Nordstrom graduated from University College London with a prize-winning degree in medicine and a first-class honours degree in neuroscience. He undertook medical training in London before starting specialist training in anaesthetics and critical care. Christopher has been involved in medical education for over eight years and has received written praise for his teaching from hospitals and universities, including Imperial College London and University College London. His academic achievements include publications in world-renowned journals, published original research and regular presentations at national and international conferences. He is one of the UK's leading UKCAT and BMAT tutors, regularly speaking at national events including the Royal Society of Medicine's Career Day and the Futurewise Careers Day.

George Rendel graduated from the University of Leeds with a prize-winning, first-class degree in English. He has used his academic understanding of the English language and his experience in journalism and publishing to become a leading expert in the verbal reasoning and essay-writing components of the UKCAT and BMAT examinations. He has worked in educational publishing for Pearson and in consulting for Accenture.

Dr Ricardo Tavares completed his prize-winning Medical Sciences Masters undergraduate degree at Oxford University and went on to finish his medical MBBS training at University College London Medical School. He carried out his foundation training within the Imperial College Deanery before starting specialist registrar training in radiology. Ricardo has several years of experience teaching medicine, both as part of a select group at Imperial College and as a clinical methods teaching tutor for Imperial College medical students. He has been published in leading international journals, spoken at numerous national conferences, and teaches on the clinical MD programme for the University of Buckingham Internal Medicine degree.

Introduction

Background

The United Kingdom Clinical Aptitude Test (UKCAT) was first introduced in 2006. Since its introduction, it has been widely used by medical and dental schools across the UK to aid in the selection of future doctors and dentists. Unlike the traditional A-Level and International Baccalaureate examinations, the UKCAT tests *aptitude*, rather than knowledge. By focusing on innate skills, it is designed to reduce the inequality which may arise between applicants from different backgrounds. This helps to widen access into medicine and dentistry.

The UKCAT consists of a two-hour computerized test. This can be sat in Test Centres across the UK. For international applicants, there are now official Test Centres in 89 countries, ensuring almost all candidates have easy access to a Test Centre.

You can choose when you sit the examination. Testing dates are available from July to the start of October, annually. Each student who takes the examination during this three-month window will get a different combination of questions. This prevents students who sit the examination later from finding out which questions will come up.

Top Tip: We recommend booking your test early, even if you wish to sit it at the end of summer, as test dates fill up quickly and the price increases.

The UKCAT examination consists of five sections, each testing a different skill set. These sections are:

- Verbal Reasoning (VR)
- Quantitative Reasoning (QR)
- Abstract Reasoning (AR)
- Decision Analysis (DA)
- Situational Judgement Test (SJT)

The Verbal and Quantitative Reasoning sections are logical tests. They assess a candidate's ability to evaluate, problem-solve and draw conclusions, based on written and numerical information.

Abstract Reasoning tests both spatial awareness and pattern recognition. This helps to identify your aptitude for constantly developing and modifying hypotheses. Decision Analysis, meanwhile, introduces complex information and tests your skills of logic and reasoning in the face of uncertainty.

The newest section of the UKCAT, Situational Judgement, was introduced in 2013. It focuses on presenting students with real-world situations and dilemmas. These are designed to identify how you react in challenging circumstances.

Booking Your Test

The UKCAT is not sat in schools or colleges, but at regional Test Centres. As such, it is down to you to book a test date in a suitable location. Initially, you will need to register online for the test and registration opens two months before the first test date. Through the online system you can book, reschedule or cancel your appointment. The price varies depending on the date you choose. In 2014, dates in July and August cost £60; subsequent dates cost £80. The price at international Test Centres outside the UK is higher and the number of available testing dates more restricted.

> **Top Tip:** Book your test date early in the summer and ensure you have two clear weeks before that date for revision. That way, if you are ill or need to reschedule, there is time to spare.

The Test Day

It is essential that you arrive at least 15 minutes before the start of your test. This will ensure you register in good time. In addition, if you rush to get there, you will add unnecessary stress to an already tough day.

You need to bring photographic identification with you. Once inside, you will be issued a permanent marker pen and laminated booklet. If you require more space to write you can ask for a supplementary booklet. If you are noise sensitive, they can provide you with earplugs at the Test Centre.

You are not allowed to bring any personal items into the examination. This includes sweets, drinks and lucky mascots! Everything you need will be provided. Once the test has started, you cannot pause or stop the test. If you need a toilet break, this will eat into your test time.

General Exam Format

The test is conducted entirely on the computers provided. The laminated booklets provided are used for calculations and making notes, and will be collected in at the end, although they will not contribute to your score. The screen is formatted so that the information for each question – text, graphs, tables etc. – is presented on the left-hand side of the screen, with the questions themselves on the right-hand side.

Once you have selected an answer, you will click the relevant option, and then the 'next' button to move to the next question. If you are unsure about an answer, you can click on the 'flag' icon to mark it for later. When you reach the end of a section, you have the option to review all questions. There is also a 'review flagged questions' button. This allows you to scroll through only those questions that you have flagged and allows you to use any remaining time efficiently on questions you were unsure about.

Top Tip: Time is your greatest enemy in the UKCAT. Use the 'flag' button sparingly and wisely to ensure you can quickly scroll through only the questions you were unsure about.

You will have a set amount of time for each question. Once your time is up you will automatically be moved on to the next section. Even if you finish another section early, you cannot go back to a previous section.

Most candidates find the time pressure the hardest part of the UKCAT exam. It is therefore essential that when you practice, you do so to time. There is an extended time version of the UKCAT available if you suffer from dyslexia: the United Kingdom Clinical Aptitude Test Special Educational Needs (UKCATSEN). The UKCATSEN is 150 minutes long, compared to 120 minutes for the standard test.

Scoring

The scoring system used in the UKCAT is complicated. The VR, QR, AR and DA sections are each scored between 300 and 900 points. Although each question is worth one mark, the raw scores are scaled to generate a score that is comparable between sections. Situational Judgement is scored differently, with more than one answer potentially scoring marks. For this section, each question is given a 'band' score, ranging from Band 1 (the best) to Band 4 (the worst).

Each section consists of a number of multiple choice questions, with between three and five answer options to choose from. There is no negative marking in any section, so it is essential that you never leave a question unanswered. Even if you do not know the correct answer, you may still guess correctly! In each chapter, we will look at how, if in doubt, you can improve your chances of getting the correct answer by logically eliminating some of the options.

Top Tip: There is no negative marking, so NEVER leave any question unanswered.

You will be presented with a printout of your scores before leaving the Test Centre. This document will contain your personal details along with your scores for each section. Once your Universities and Colleges Admissions Services (UCAS) application is complete, your chosen universities will automatically be notified of your results. You do not need to send them any additional information.

You can only sit the UKCAT examination once per academic year. Your score is valid for entry to university programmes starting the following academic year (unless you have applied for deferred entry, in which case it is valid for your deferred start date). Unfortunately, if you do not do well at the exam you will need to wait a full year before you can re-sit.

Most universities take the UKCAT into account but they do so in different ways. This can vary from year to year, so it is essential that you read the latest information on university websites and prospectuses.

Some universities look at certain subsections of the test more closely than others. Some look at the overall score. Some universities have minimum cut-offs, or averages, that you must meet in order to apply. At certain institutions, your UKCAT score will only make up part of your application score; the remaining points will come from your personal statement and A-Level results. Others give out invitations to interview based entirely on UKCAT scores.

Below is a table showing how the scores varied between 2013 and 2014:

	2013	2014
Verbal Reasoning	557	571
Quantitative Reasoning	655	684
Abstract Reasoning	661	636
Decision Analysis	771	614
Total	2643	2505
Average	661	626

There was a considerable drop in total scores between 2013 and 2014, with the average total score falling by almost 150 points. Although the score in most sections remained similar, it was in Decision Analysis where the largest change arose.

> **Top Tip:** The last UKCAT testing date is two weeks before the UCAS submission date. Apply to universities where your score will benefit your application the most. For instance, if your score isn't as high as you had hoped, then apply to universities which do not focus heavily on UKCAT scores.

General Technique

Although the UKCAT is an aptitude test, it is well documented that you can significantly boost your score through practice. In this book we will cover specific techniques that you can apply in order to excel in each section. In addition, there are some general techniques that are applicable to all sections.

Every year, general feedback shows that timing is the biggest challenge. The exam is intense. It requires considerable mental stamina to keep the momentum going for the full two hours. It is therefore essential that you 'train' regularly – just like you would for a marathon. In the run up to the exam you should have a structured revision plan, devoting set amounts of time to regular practice. In addition to doing practice questions, you should do timed mock exams that simulate the real exam as much as possible.

When you start doing practice questions it is useful to allow yourself extra time for each question. Once you develop your skills and understand the format you should begin to reduce the time you allocate yourself per question. Eventually, you will complete all questions within the time allowed. By doing questions to time you will ensure that you are as prepared as possible for the test.

As there is no negative marking you must never leave an answer blank. Even if you do not know how to answer a question, there are ways to help improve your odds beyond that of simply guessing. This is a concept that we will develop in later chapters. A blank answer guarantees a score of 0 on that question. An educated guess, on the other hand, provides you with a 1 in 2–5 chance of success (depending on the question type).

General Top Tips

- Always practice questions to time.
- Try to simulate the exam conditions when practising (e.g. do not take breaks, have drinks etc.).
- Understand and use the flag button to ensure you can quickly review questions which you were unsure about.
- Never leave a question blank; there is no negative marking.
- If you are stuck on a question then put down an answer, flag the question and move on.
- Practice allows you to significantly boost your score; set up a structured, intense revision plan two weeks before the exam – and stick to it!
- The exam is tough, so make sure you're well rested the night before and arrive with plenty of time to spare to avoid unnecessary stress.

CHAPTER 1

Verbal Reasoning

Overview

As a doctor, you are committing to a lifetime of learning. This will include regularly reading medical journals, picking out crucial information and deciding how to modify your practice based on the latest evidence.

There will also be times when you will need to assess critical situations and pick out the key factors in a short space of time. The Verbal Reasoning section of the UKCAT tests your ability to quickly absorb and interpret information.

Format of the Section

This section consists of 11 **Question Sets**. These are each made up of a 200–400 word passage and four associated questions, or **Items**.

There are two different types of Question Sets:

1. True, False, Can't Tell

   Each Item is a short statement. Your task is to say, based purely on the passage provided, whether the statement is 'True' or 'False', or if you 'Can't Tell' whether it is true or false, based on the information given.

2. Free Text

   Items can be incomplete statements or short questions. Rather than three set answer options – as with 'True', 'False' or 'Can't Tell' – you are given four 'free text' options and must choose one.

You have 22 minutes to complete the Verbal Reasoning section. This means that you will only have 2 minutes per Question Set, or 30 seconds per Item.

The time pressure is intense. That is why you need to go into this section with a well-rehearsed strategy.

Logically Follows

Regardless of the Question Set format, it is imperative that your answer reflects only what *logically follows* from the passage. If something 'logically follows' from the passage, you can't help but reach the conclusion offered, based on the passage alone, without any assumptions or outside knowledge.

Core Strategy

You can't afford to read the whole passage thoroughly and then address each Item. There simply isn't time! So, when you start a Question Set, leave the passage unread and go straight to the first Item.

The fundamental strategy you should then employ, regardless of the Question Set type, involves six simple steps:

1. Read the statement/incomplete statement/question

2. Skim the passage for key words and phrases relating to this

3. Read the sentence(s) containing the key words, as well as those before and after

4. Continue scanning the passage for further occurrences of the key words

5. If found again, repeat step 3

6. Select an answer based on this 'targeted' reading

These six steps should be repeated for each Item.

That is the bedrock of your approach. Stick to it, and you will put yourself in a strong position to complete the section in time, and start building a respectable score.

To excel, you should tinker your technique according to the **Question Set Format**, develop an understanding of **Clue Words** and what they signify, and recognise the **Common Tricks** that question writers use.

'True', 'False' or 'Can't Tell'

In order to tackle the 'True', 'False' or 'Can't Tell' Question Sets effectively, your understanding of each of those three terms must be crystal clear:

True: On the basis of the information in the passage, it logically follows that the statement is true.

False: On the basis of the information in the passage, it logically follows that the statement is false.

Can't Tell: You cannot tell from the information in the passage whether the statement is true or false.

Clue Words

Verbal Reasoning questions are not created by a computer. They are written by human beings. Understanding this point – and taking a few seconds to put yourself in the shoes of the question writer – can often help you reach the correct solution.

In order to make each statement fit neatly into just one of the three options – 'True', 'False' or 'Can't Tell' – the question writer has to use words that specifically signpost one of those three answers, or that discount the other two.

The vocabulary available to help them do this is quite limited. Therefore, certain words can act as 'clues' as to what the answer might – or might not – be.

There are two types of 'clue' words that are particularly significant:

1. Definitive Words – Definitive Words are those that help make a statement 'black and white'. They tend to shut down multiple possibilities, and leave us with only one viable option. These include: 'impossible'; 'cannot'; 'never'; 'only'; 'solely'; 'certainly'; 'exclusively'; 'must'; 'always'.

    For example, the statement 'Ferraris are only red' leaves no room for doubt as to what colour a Ferrari is.

2. Mitigating Words – Mitigating Words are those that make a statement less definitive and introduce 'shades of grey'. They tend to open up multiple possibilities. These include: 'might'; 'could'; 'can'; 'sometimes'; 'often'; 'frequently'; 'likely'; 'rarely'.

    For example, the statement 'Ferraris are *sometimes* red' opens up the possibility that Ferraris could be blue, black, silver etc.

These 'clue' words won't automatically give you the right answer. But they should act as red flags, and prompt you to ask yourself: *Why has the question writer included these words in the statement, or in the relevant part of the passage?*

They are not there by mistake; they are serving a purpose. Therefore, you should view them as signposts to guide you towards the right answer. Often, it is the presence of these words that will ultimately signal whether the answer is 'True', 'False' or 'Can't Tell'.

On the surface, Mitigating Words lend themselves more to 'Can't Tell', while Definitive Words lean towards 'True' or 'False'.

But more important is whether the *type* of 'clue' words – definitive or mitigating – in the statement, match those in the corresponding part of the passage.

Example 1

The statement is definitive, but the relevant part of the passage is mitigated. Or the statement is mitigated, but the relevant part of the passage is definitive. This **mismatch** often means that the likely answer is either 'False' or 'Can't Tell'.

Statement: Ferrari *never* makes blue cars [definitive].

Relevant part of passage: Ferrari *usually* makes red cars [mitigated].

Answer: Can't Tell

Example 2

If the statement and the relevant part of the passage are *both* either definitive or mitigated, this **match** often lends itself to a 'True' or 'False' answer.

Statement: Ferrari *solely* makes red cars [definitive].

Relevant part of passage: Ferrari *never* makes cars that are not red [definitive].

Answer: True

Top Tip: Look out for definitive and mitigating 'clue' words. Ask yourself why the question writer included them. Check if the type of 'clue' words in the statement and the passage match.

Common Tricks

In the Verbal Reasoning section, there are a number of 'tricks' that question writers can use to catch you out. Over the next few pages, we are going to demonstrate these through example questions.

Each question will use a common 'trick'. Do your best to answer all questions within each set, before reading the explanations. Once you are aware of the main 'tricks', and the mechanics of how they work, you will quickly learn how to recognise and overcome them in exam situations.

Refer to **Example Set 1**, below. Using the **six-step strategy**, and looking out for **clue words**, answer all four questions in **2 minutes**. Make a note of your answers before moving on to the explanations.

Example Set 1

Scientology is a body of beliefs and practices, started in 1952 by science fiction writer L Ron Hubbard. Hubbard was succeeded by the current leader of Scientology, David Miscavige, in 1987.

The Church of Scientology was granted tax exemption by the US Internal Revenue Service in 1993, on this basis that it was a 'religion'. Scientology is also recognised as a religion by countries including Sweden, Spain and Portugal. However, other nations, like Canada and the United Kingdom, do not afford Scientology religious recognition. Many people go as far as to suggest that it is a cult, and, moreover, that it brainwashes and extorts money from its followers. This might be because it is impossible to ascend the ranks of the Church of Scientology without paying cash to advance through the various levels, which range from 'Clear' to Operating Thetan Levels I through XV.

It can be widely read on the Internet (which practising Scientologists are deterred from using), that Scientology scriptures make reference to a character named Xenu. As dictator of the 'Galactic Confederacy', Xenu supposedly brought billions of his people to Earth 75 million years ago, stacked them around volcanoes and killed them using hydrogen bombs. Some ex-Scientologists have said that the Church of Scientology only tells its followers about Xenu when they reach Operating Thetan Level III.

Perhaps the most famous practitioner of Scientology is Tom Cruise, who is an Operating Thetan Level VII. David Miscavige was Tom Cruise's best man at his wedding to Katie Holmes in 2006. Cruise has spoken in favour of the Church of Scientology many times since joining it in 1990.

1. The leader of Scientology was Tom Cruise's best man in his marriage to Katie Holmes.

    A.   True

    B.   False

    C.   Can't Tell

2. Tom Cruise has been told about Xenu by the Church of Scientology.

    A.   True

    B.   False

    C.   Can't Tell

3. The Church of Scientology is not exempt from paying taxes in Canada and the UK.

    A.   True

    B.   False

    C.   Can't Tell

4. Actor Tom Cruise is arguably the most famous practitioner of Scientology.

    A.   True

    B.   False

    C.   Can't Tell

Example Set 1: Answers and Explanations

Question 1

The leader of Scientology was Tom Cruise's best man in his marriage to Katie Holmes.

ANSWER: True

We know from the last paragraph that David Miscavige was Tom Cruise's best man at his wedding to Katie Holmes in 2006. We also know from the first paragraph that David Miscavige is the current leader of Scientology, and has been since succeeding L Ron Hubbard in 1987.

This question is a demonstration of **Dispersion of Key Words**.

Dispersion of Key Words

Question writers know you will be scanning the passage for the key word(s) from the statement. This is a common strategy. When there is only one mention of the key word(s) in the passage, it makes life easier. But question writers don't always want your life to be easy! So they sometimes make things harder, ensuring that:

1. The same key word/phrase is used in different places throughout the passage; or

2. Different keys words/phrases from the statement are scattered throughout the passage

In this example, the key words are 'David Miscavige'. Scanning for this set of words, we see that it is mentioned in the second sentence. However, it is important to **keep scanning** for all mentions of the key word throughout the passage. Otherwise, we might miss crucial information that confirms, mitigates or, as in this case, elaborates on the information we already have.

Example Set 1: Answers and Explanations

Question 2

Tom Cruise has been told about Xenu by the Church of Scientology.

ANSWER: Can't Tell

From the third paragraph, we know that 'some ex-Scientologists' have said that the Church of Scientology tells its followers about Xenu at Operating Thetan Level III. Tom Cruise is an Operating Thetan Level VII. So, if the ex-Scientologists referred to are telling the truth, then Tom Cruise would have been told about Xenu by the Church of Scientology.

However, in the phrase '*some* ex-Scientologists', the word 'some' is a clear mitigation. We cannot assume that something is true, just because 'some' people have said it. Furthermore, the fact that we are only told what has been said, rather than what definitively *is*, represents a further form of mitigation, confirming that the correct answer is 'Can't Tell'.

This question is a demonstration of **Mitigation**.

Mitigation and Contradiction

Mitigation and contradiction occurs when one part of the passage appears to confirm the statement as true or false, only for another part of the passage to provide further information which challenges this.

Mitigation or contradiction can occur within the same sentence as the key word(s) from the statement. But sometimes mitigation or contradiction comes in the sentence before or after. So, make sure that you scan the sentences that precede and follow the one containing your key word(s) – just in case! If mitigation or contradiction occurs elsewhere in the passage, hopefully your search for dispersed key word(s) will lead you to it.

Example Set 1: Answers and Explanations

Question 3

The Church of Scientology is not exempt from paying taxes in Canada and the UK.

ANSWER: Can't Tell

We know that the Church of Scientology is exempt from paying taxes in the United States because the Internal Revenue Service recognises it as a religion. We know that the UK and Canada do not recognise it as a religion, but this does not prohibit it being exempt from paying taxes in those countries for some other reason.

This question is a demonstration of **Faulty Logic**.

Faulty Logic

Faulty logic occurs when the *structure* of the argument employed does not make logical sense. This can lead to reasonable premises – in terms of content – being used to justify an unsound conclusion. There are some common examples of faulty logic that tend to recur in the Verbal Reasoning section of the UKCAT. A key piece of logic to remember is: *If X means Y, then Y does not necessarily mean X.*

Example: All humans are mammals, but not all mammals are human.

Causation

Causation is another logic-related pitfall. So, whenever causation comes up, that should act as a red flag. The question writer will often try to tempt you into *assuming* a causal relationship between two things in the passage, where such a relationship does not logically follow.

Example: Saying that many people who eat a lot of chocolate suffer frequent headaches is not the same as saying that eating chocolate causes headaches!

Top Tip: Remember: Just because many people who do X also do/have/are Y, we cannot assume that X causes Y (unless stated explicitly in the passage).

Example Set 1: Answers and Explanations

Question 4

Actor Tom Cruise is arguably the most famous practitioner of Scientology.

ANSWER: Can't Tell

In the final paragraph, we read that: 'perhaps the most famous practitioner of Scientology is Tom Cruise'. This appears to corroborate the statement. However, nowhere in the passage are we told that Tom Cruise is an 'actor'. Nor is the possibility excluded. So we cannot tell, from the information given, whether or not the statement is true or false.

This question is a demonstration of **Outside Knowledge**.

Outside Knowledge

You should NEVER bring outside knowledge into your reasoning. Remember: *It is important to base your answer only on the information in the passage and not on any other knowledge you may have.*

Question writers might try to trick you into using outside knowledge. They can do this by throwing in something that you will almost certainly know, but that does not follow logically from the passage. In the above example, you will know that Tom Cruise is an actor, but it is not stated in the passage and is not a logical inference.

Another way to lure you into using outside knowledge is to appeal to your ego. If you have good general knowledge, it's natural to want to show this off. For instance, if you are told that a vessel was travelling at 770 miles/hour, you might be tempted to say it is 'true' that the vessel in question broke the speed barrier. But unless we are explicitly told in the passage that this happened, or that the speed barrier is 768 miles/hour, the actual answer would be 'Can't Tell'.

> **Top Tip:** If the statement refers to something you know, but it is not explicitly stated within the passage, don't fall for it!

To demonstrate the next common 'tricks' we're going to use a different passage. Please refer to **Example Set 2**, below. As before, use the **six-step strategy** and look out for **clue words**. There are only two questions in this set, so you have just **1 minute** to finish both. Make a note of your answers to all questions before moving on to the explanations.

Example Set 2

Lance Armstrong was one of the world's most celebrated sportsmen, having won seven consecutive Tour de France races between 1999 and 2005. This feat was all the more remarkable as it came after he was diagnosed with advanced testicular cancer in 1996. Armstrong undeniably achieved things that have never been matched before or since, and was respected as much for his work off the bike as on it. In 1997, he launched the Lance Armstrong Foundation to provide support to cancer sufferers. The name of the foundation was changed to Livestrong in 2003.

Rumours had long circulated that Armstrong might have been involved with doping. These rumours had always been fiercely rebuffed by Armstrong and his representatives. For example, he successfully sued the *Sunday Times* and its writer David Walsh for alleging that he had cheated during his Tour successes. However, in 2012 Armstrong was banned from cycling for life by the United States Anti-Doping Agency (USADA). He was also accused of running 'the most sophisticated, professionalized and successful doping program that sport has ever seen'.

After initial protestations, Armstrong admitted to taking banned substances when he appeared on the *Oprah Winfrey Show* in January 2013. There were a number of legal consequences to this admission. Among others, Armstrong was sued by SCA Promotions for the $12 million it paid out insuring his Tour wins, and was also counter-sued by the *Sunday Times*.

1. Armstrong's achievements were unique.

   A.   True

   B.   False

   C.   Can't Tell

2. USADA accused Armstrong of running 'the most sophisticated, professionalized and successful doping program that sport has ever seen'.

   A.   True

   B.   False

   C.   Can't Tell

Example Set 2: Answers and Explanations

Question 1

Armstrong's achievements were unique.

ANSWER: True

The word 'unique' does not arise in the passage. However, we are told that Armstrong 'undeniably achieved things that have never been matched before or since'. The fact that this is 'undeniable' means that it is certain. And saying that his achievements have 'never been matched before or since' is effectively synonymous with saying that they were 'unique'.

This question is a demonstration of **Synonyms**.

Synonyms

We have already examined the way question writers can make the 'skimming' strategy more challenging by **Dispersion of Key Words and Phrases** throughout the passage.

Another even trickier technique they can employ to throw you off is to use synonymous words or phrases in the passage, rather than the precise ones from the statement. This means that you can't simply look for the same word; you also need to be aware of words which mean the same thing. Since this requires more interpretation, it becomes a more difficult task.

Usually, you won't have to worry as there will be some identical vocabulary from the statement to signal the relevant part of the passage. This will give you the foothold you need to ensure you are in the right place. But, just occasionally, that won't be the case. Ultimately, this means that you have to look for both:

1. Key words/phrases

   and

2. Synonymous key words/phrases

Of course, you will not be able to think of *all* synonymous words and phrases and skim the passage looking for them. That wouldn't be very time efficient at all. But what you can do is take a mental note of words or expressions that have a similar meaning. If you don't find the specific word in question, then these similar words/expressions will be your next port of call.

> **Top Tip:** You can also use other key words as a guide. In the example above, looking for 'achievements' will take you to 'achieved'. By reading around this, you will notice that the subsequent wording makes clear that the achievements referred to were unique.

Example Set 2: Answers and Explanations

Question 2

USADA accused Armstrong of running 'the most sophisticated, professionalized and successful doping program that sport has ever seen'.

ANSWER: Can't Tell

Reference to USADA is made in the second paragraph. We are told that they banned Armstrong from cycling for life in 2012. The next sentence has the crucial quote about 'running the most sophisticated, professionalized and successful doping program that sport has ever seen'. But, while USADA is mentioned in the preceding sentence, these words are not attributed to USADA. Nor are they attributed to anyone else. Therefore, we can't tell if they came from USADA or not.

This question is a demonstration of **Juxtaposition**.

Juxtaposition

Juxtaposition occurs when two ideas or objects are placed next to each other within the passage. The key thing to remember is that just because two things are stated in close proximity, it does not mean that they are linked – even if they refer to similar topics and use similar language.

Question writers will often include two statements side by side, hoping that you will *assume* a link between them that is not explicitly stated and does not logically follow from the passage. In order to avoid this pitfall, there are some simple dos and don'ts that you should adhere to:

Do – Look for **bridging phrases**. These are short phrases that suggest a genuine and explicit link between two pieces of information. They include: 'because of'; 'due to'; and 'as a result of'. When you see these or similar phrases they often suggest a link and/or a causal relationship between two things.

Do not – *Assume* that two statements are linked, or have a causal relationship. That they relate to the same theme is not enough. In order to logically infer a link and/or a causal relationship, the passage must make the link explicit – usually by employing a **bridging phrase**.

Recall our example of assumed causation when we discussed **Faulty Logic**: *Saying that many people who eat a lot of chocolate suffer frequent headaches is not the same as saying that eating chocolate causes headaches!*

Read the following statement: *Chocolate causes headaches.* Now, consider whether that statement is 'True', 'False' or if you 'Can't Tell', based first on Sample 1 and then on Sample 2.

Sample 1

A study was conducted into people who suffer an above-average amount of headaches. These people were given a survey about their life style. The survey showed that they also ate an above-average amount of chocolate.

Chocolate causes headaches.

   A. True

   B. False

   C. Can't Tell

Sample 2

A study was conducted into people who suffer an above-average amount of headaches. These people were given a survey about their life style. A scientific experiment proved that the frequency of their headaches was a result of the fact they also ate an above-average amount of chocolate.

Chocolate causes headaches.

   A. True

   B. False

   C. Can't Tell

Answer Sample 1: Can't Tell

Though we are told that the people who suffered an above-average number of headaches also ate an above-average amount of chocolate, there is nothing to logically infer a link between the two. We can't assume that chocolate causes the headaches, because there could be any number of other factors involved. The chocolate could be a mere coincidence. There are no bridging phrases linking the two things or establishing a causal relationship.

Answer Sample 2: True

In this case, we have a clear bridging phrase – 'was a result of' – that establishes a causal relationship between the chocolate and the headaches. We also have definitive language: this relationship was 'proved'.

> **Top Tip:** Look for **bridging phrases** that signal a causal relationship. Don't assume links/causal relationships based on juxtaposition!

To demonstrate the next common 'tricks' we're going to use a different passage. Please refer to **Example Set 3**, below. As before, use the **six-step strategy** and look out for **clue words**. There are only two questions in this set, so you have just **1 minute** to finish both. Make a note of your answers to all questions before moving on to the explanations.

Example Set 3

Amanda Knox served 4 years in prison in Italy for the murder of Meredith Kercher in Perugia in 2007. The trial was covered extensively by media around the world. There are many reasons for this, including the unusual and macabre nature of the murder of the young English student. But the centre of attention was undeniably Knox herself, whose youth, good looks and often strange behaviour before and during the murder trial made her both famous and infamous. Also convicted of the murder was Knox's then boyfriend, Raffaele Sollecito, who was given a 25-year sentence – one year less than Knox.

Knox and her legal team had always pointed to a number of inconsistencies in the case against her. The defence repeatedly cited the possible contamination of DNA evidence used against her, as well as her treatment during questioning. This was allegedly aggressive and conducted over many consecutive hours in Italian: a language that Knox did not then understand fluently. In 2009, her family told the *Sunday Times* that Knox had not been given an interpreter.

Knox and Sollecito's convictions were overturned on October 3, 2011, after a second appeal. The decision was based largely on a 145-page report questioning the validity of the DNA evidence. The hearing was conducted solely in Italian, and Knox spoke in detail, clearly and cohesively, when called upon. After being released, Knox returned to the United States, where she lives with her family. However, her acquittal was overturned in March 2013, and the case will go back to court. If she is found guilty, the Italian authorities could demand her extradition from the United States.

1. Amanda Knox speaks Italian well.

   A.   True

   B.   False

   C.   Can't Tell

2. Amanda Knox was given a sentence of at least 26 years.

   A.   True

   B.   False

   C.   Can't Tell

Example Set 3: Answers and Explanations

Question 1

Amanda Knox speaks Italian well.

ANSWER: True

In the third paragraph, we are told that: 'The hearing was conducted solely in Italian, and Knox spoke in detail, clearly and cohesively, when called upon.' The key word is 'solely'. If the only language spoken was Italian and Knox was able to speak in detail, with clarity and cohesion, it is fair to infer that she speaks Italian well.

There is a red herring in the second paragraph, when reference is made to her being questioned in a language 'Knox did not then understand fluently'. The key mitigating word is 'then', making the statement historical. It is superseded by the information in the last paragraph.

This question is a demonstration of a statement that **Sounds Like Can't Tell** (but isn't!).

Sounds Like Can't Tell

There are a couple of sneaky ways of making a statement seem like an obvious 'Can't Tell' when, in fact, it is 'True' or 'False'. This includes the absence, from the statement, passage or both, of key words, combined with the use of subjective words that seem like they will be hard to confirm or refute.

We can combat the absence of key words by being particularly vigilant for **Synonyms** – those words and phrases that mean the same as something in the statement, even if the vocabulary is not identical.

Using subjective terms primes us to select a 'Can't Tell' answer. In the above example, one may think: 'how do you define speaking Italian "well"?' We might think that this is not possible, and quickly guess at 'Can't Tell'. But, as shown by the explanation, it is possible to make a **value judgement** from logical inference.

Example Set 3: Answers and Explanations

Question 2

Amanda Knox was given a sentence of at least 26 years.

ANSWER: False

We know from the end of the first paragraph that Raffaele Sollecito was given a 25-year sentence and that this was 'one less than Knox'. We can therefore calculate, from the information given, that Amanda was given a sentence of exactly 26 years. To say the sentence was 'at least 26 years' is therefore false.

This is an example of statements that use **Numbers**.

Numbers

Basic calculations are a form of logical inference, so be prepared to do quick additions, subtractions and multiplications in your head to arrive at the right answer. For example: *In the kitchen, there are two apples in the fruit bowl and two apples in the fridge, and no apples anywhere else.* Based on this information, it would be 'true' to say that there are four apples in the kitchen, as this does follow logically from the passage.

Averages

Averages come up quite frequently in the Verbal Reasoning section. There is a trick associated with averages that can be explained through the following example: You are told that the average height of boys in a sixth form class is 170 centimetres. You might, therefore, assume that it is 'true' that some boys are shorter and some taller than 170 cm. However, it is *possible* (unless specifically discounted) that *all* the boys are exactly 170 cm. So the answer to the statement: 'one or more boys are shorter/taller than 170 cm' is actually 'Can't Tell'.

> **Top Tip:** When an average is given, remember that, as well as numbers below and above, there might be numbers that are **exactly equal** to this average.

Summary of Common Tricks

1. Dispersion of Key Words

2. Mitigation and Contradiction

3. Faulty Logic

4. Outside Knowledge

5. Juxtaposition

6. Synonyms

7. Sounds Like 'Can't Tell'

8. Numbers and Averages

Free Text Question Sets

'Free Text' Question Sets were introduced in 2013. They now make up a significant percentage of the Verbal Reasoning section. In fact, in recent years, they outnumbered the 'True', 'False' or 'Can't Tell' questions.

It is first worth noting what is the same and what is different in the 'Free Text' format.

What's the Same?

- The Passage – same length and topic types
- Number of Items per passage – still four
- Key principles – still what 'logically follows'
- Common Tricks – same ones … plus a few more!

What's Different?

True, False, Can't Tell	Free Text
Items are complete statements	Items are incomplete statements/questions
3 answer options	4 answer options
Always 'True', 'False' or 'Can't Tell'	Possible answers are free text
Time pressured	Even more time pressured!

Strategy

You can still follow the core six-step strategy. However, there are some nuances you can add to improve results for this format:

1. Skim passage for the key words/phrases from the question/incomplete statement

2. Read around those key words/phrases to gain a high level sense of what the passage has to say on that topic

3. Read the answer options one by one, cross-referencing against the relevant part of the passage where needed

4. Discount non-viable options straight away

   - If you reach a perfect fit, select it and move on
   - If there is no perfect fit, assess all options and choose best

Item Types

Before 2013, when all the Items asked if the statement was 'True', 'False' or 'Can't Tell', you knew exactly what to expect. That's no longer the case. In the 'Free Text' format, each answer option can say pretty much anything. It may seem that the possibilities are endless.

However, in reality, Items within this Question Set format generally fall into one of a limited number of categories. You can be asked to identify:

- The correct ending to incomplete statements
- Whether something is true/false
- Conclusions/definitions from the passage
- Causes/consequences of certain things

And though they might try to muddy the water by asking you to make Value Judgements, your strategy will largely remain the same.

We are now going to tackle each of these Item categories with some more worked-through examples.

Please refer to **Example Set 4**, below. The passage is similar to the one used in **Example Set 3**, but there are key differences so be careful! There is only one question in this set, so try to answer in **30 seconds**.

Example Set 4

Amanda Knox served 4 years in prison in Italy for the murder of Meredith Kercher in Perugia in 2007. The trial was covered extensively by media around the world. There are many reasons for this, including the unusual and macabre nature of the murder of the young English student. But the centre of attention was undeniably Knox herself, whose youth, good looks and often strange behaviour before and during the murder trial made her both famous and infamous. Also convicted of the murder was Knox's then boyfriend, Raffaele Sollecito, who was given a 25-year sentence – one year less than Knox.

Knox and her legal team had always pointed to a number of inconsistencies in the case against her. The defence repeatedly cited the possible contamination of DNA evidence used against her, as well as her treatment during questioning. This was allegedly aggressive, and conducted over many consecutive hours in Italian: a language that Knox did not then understand fluently. In 2009, her family told the *Sunday Times* that Knox had not been given an interpreter.

Knox and Sollecito's convictions were overturned on October 3, 2011, after a second appeal. The decision was based largely on a 145-page report questioning the validity of the DNA evidence. The hearing was conducted solely in Italian, and Knox spoke in detail, clearly and cohesively, when called upon. After being released, Knox returned to the United States, where she lives with her family. However, her acquittal was overturned in March 2013, and the case will go back to court. If she is found guilty, the Italian authorities could demand her extradition from the United States.

1. Knox's conviction was overturned mainly because:

    A.   The trial was a centre of media attention around the world.

    B.   She was treated aggressively when questioned.

    C.   The DNA evidence was false.

    D.   A report raised questions about some of the evidence.

Example Set 4: Answers and Explanations

Question 1

Knox's conviction was overturned mainly because ...

ANSWER: D

The key part of the passage is: 'Knox and Sollecito's convictions were overturned on October 3, 2011, after a second appeal. The decision was based largely on a 145-page report questioning the validity of the DNA evidence.'

Since the decision to overturn was based 'largely' on this report we know that the report was the main reason. Since it questions the validity of the DNA evidence, it clearly questioned the evidence. And since it was significant enough to get the decision overturned, we can also infer that the evidence was 'key'.

This an example of an **Incomplete Statement**, which is the most common Item type in the free text format.

Incomplete Statement

Often, you will be presented with incomplete sentences and asked to select the right ending. For example:

* 'Mercury has not been extensively studied because ...'
* 'Poverty is a relative measure because ...'

When faced with this format, you should treat each answer option as a mini 'True', 'False' or 'Can't Tell' task.

Only if the complete sentence – i.e. the partial statement ending with the given answer option – is 'True', is that answer correct.

Please refer to **Example Set 5**, below. The passage will be familiar – but the questions won't be! There are four questions in this set, so you have **2 minutes** to finish. Make a note of your answers to all questions before moving on to the explanations.

Example Set 5

Scientology is a body of beliefs and practices, started in 1952 by science fiction writer L Ron Hubbard. Hubbard was succeeded by the current leader of Scientology, David Miscavige, in 1987.

The Church of Scientology was granted tax exemption by the US Internal Revenue Service in 1993, on this basis that it was a 'religion'. Scientology is also recognised as a religion by countries including Sweden, Spain and Portugal. However, other nations, like Canada and the United Kingdom, do not afford Scientology religious recognition. Many people go as far as to suggest that it is a cult, and, moreover, that it brainwashes and extorts money from its followers. This might be because it is impossible to ascend the ranks of the Church of Scientology without paying cash to advance through the various levels, which range from 'Clear' to Operating Thetan Levels I through XV.

It can be widely read on the Internet (which practising Scientologists are deterred from using), that Scientology scriptures make reference to a character named Xenu. As dictator of the 'Galactic Confederacy', Xenu supposedly brought billions of his people to Earth 75 million years ago, stacked them around volcanoes and killed them using hydrogen bombs. Some ex-Scientologists have said that the Church of Scientology only tells its followers about Xenu when they reach Operating Thetan Level III.

Perhaps the most famous practitioner of Scientology is Tom Cruise, who is an Operating Thetan Level VII. David Miscavige was Tom Cruise's best man at his wedding to Katie Holmes in 2006. Cruise has spoken in favour of the Church of Scientology many times since joining it in 1990.

1. If the passage is true, which of the following statements is also true?

    A. Tom Cruise has paid money to the Church of Scientology.

    B. L Ron Hubbard died in 1987.

    C. There are many Scientologists in Spain.

    D. Canada and the UK have the same tax system.

2. Based on the passage, which of the following statements is most likely to be true?

    A. David Miscavige is related to L Ron Hubbard.

    B. Reference to Xenu is easily found online.

    C. Scientologists never go on the Internet.

    D. Katie Holmes is a Scientologist.

3. Which of the following statements, if true, would weaken the argument that Scientology is a cult?

    A. Senior Scientologists claim they have not been brainwashed.

    B. Senior Scientologists have not paid any money to the Church of Scientology.

C. Scientology is granted tax exemptions in over 20 countries.

D. Scientology does not completely ban followers from using the Internet.

4. Which of the following conclusions about Scientology can be drawn from the passage?

A. Scientology is based on the science fiction of L Ron Hubbard.

B. Scientology is a cult.

C. Scientology is recognised as a religion in some countries but not others.

D. Scientology actively looks to recruit celebrity followers.

Example Set 5: Answers and Explanations

Question 1

If the passage is true, which of the following statements is also true?

ANSWER: A

Looking for key words, we learn that levels of Scientology range from 'Clear' to 'Operating Thetan Levels I through XV'. We know that Tom Cruise is an Operating Thetan Level VII. We also know that 'it is impossible to ascend the ranks of the Church of Scientology without paying cash to advance through the various levels'. Therefore, in order to have reached Operating Thetan Level VII, Tom Cruise must have given money to the Church of Scientology.

This is an example of a **Free Text True or False**.

Free Text True or False

In the free text question sets, you might still be asked whether something is true or false. When this happens, you can apply the same principles that have been established for the 'True', 'False' or 'Can't Tell' format.

Common examples:

- Which of the following is/is always true?
- If the passage is true, which of the following is also true?
- Which of the following is most/least likely to be true?

In order to find the right answer, you should employ the following strategy:

1. Use exactly the same methodology as the 'True', 'False', 'Can't Tell'.

2. It is only 'True' if it logically follows with no assumptions.

3. Treat each option like a mini 'True', 'False', 'Can't Tell' exercise.

4. Stop when you find a logically perfect answer.

Example Set 5: Answers and Explanations

Question 2

Based on the passage, which of the following statements is most likely to be true?

ANSWER: B

A. We only know that David Miscavige succeeded L Ron Hubbard as leader of Scientology. This does not mean they are related.

B. **We are told that it can be 'widely read on the Internet' that there is a character called Xenu in the Scientology Scriptures. For this to be the case, it is likely to be true that references to Xenu are common online.**

C. Though we know that Scientologists are 'deterred from using' the Internet, this does not mean they never do so.

D. We know only that Tom Cruise is a Scientologist and that his wedding to Katie Holmes was in 2006. There is nothing in this to imply she is a Scientologist herself.

This is also a free text true or false question. But it is also a **Value Judgement** question, because it asks you to make a qualitative assessment of the information when choosing an answer.

Value Judgement

Value Judgements can be introduced to any Item type.

Common examples:

- Which of the following best supports X?
- Which of the following is most/least likely to be true?
- Which of the following is the most influential cause of X?
- Which of these measures are most/least effective?
- Which of the following would strengthen/weaken X argument?
- When doing X, Y is … (e.g. good, bad, indifferent etc.).

Strategy:

1. Don't settle on an answer without assessing all options.

2. Dismiss non-viable answers and weigh up the remainder.

3. Go with best fit, even though there might be shades of grey.

Top Tip: Sometimes you will be asked about the **Author's View** on something in the passage. This is simply another way of introducing a Value Judgement, and the same rules apply.

Another Value Judgement you are often asked to make is whether something will **Strengthen or Weaken** the argument in the passage.

Example Set 5: Answers and Explanations

Question 3

Which of the following statements, if true, would weaken the argument that Scientology is a cult?

ANSWER: B

The key word in this question is 'cult'. This leads us to the line in the second paragraph: 'many people go as far as to suggest that it is a cult, on the basis that it brainwashes and extorts money from its followers'. So 'brainwashing' and 'extortion' are the keys to the argument that Scientology is cult.

Reading further, we know that the notion of 'extortion' comes from the fact that you need to pay in order to 'advance through the various levels' of Scientology. If Senior Scientologists have not paid money, however, this 'extortion' would therefore be largely disproved.

This would remove one of the key foundations to the argument that Scientology is a cult, weakening it considerably.

This is a classic **Strengthen/Weaken** question.

Strengthen/Weaken

When faced with this format, remember:

- A point **strengthens** an argument if it supports or adds to any of the premise(s) that lead to its conclusion.
- A point **weakens** an argument if it undermines the premise(s) that lead to its conclusion.

Similar to **Strengthening/Weakening** questions, you might also be asked how 'effective' something is, according to the passage.

Question: How can you judge whether something has been more or less effective than something else?

Answer: By measurable results which achieve a stated goal

Example Set 5: Answers and Explanations

Question 4

Which of the following conclusions about Scientology can be drawn from the passage?

ANSWER: C

We know that Scientology is recognised as a religion by some countries, including Sweden, Spain and Portugal. We also know that it is 'not afforded religious recognition' in the UK and Canada. We can therefore conclude that it is recognised as a religion in some countries but not others.

This is an example of a **Conclusions/Definitions** question.

Conclusions/Definitions

Common examples:

- What conclusion on X can be drawn from the passage?
- Which of the following can be inferred from the passage?
- Which statement best supports/is supported by the passage?
- What is the definition of X?

Strategy:

1. A valid conclusion is one that follows logically from the passage.
2. Therefore, a valid conclusion is exactly the same as a 'True' answer.
3. Basically, the question is asking: 'Which of the following is "True"?'
4. Again, treat each option like a 'mini' 'True', 'False' 'Can't Tell' exercise.
5. Stop when you find a logically perfect answer.

Cause and Consequence

You will often be asked about the causes and/or consequences of things in the passage. Whenever this happens, simply apply the rules established for **Causation**, explained earlier in this chapter.

In other words, never assume links between two pieces of information, even if they seem related or are juxtaposed. In order for things to be related, they require a **Bridging Phrase**.

Bridging Phrase

Common examples:

- Which of the following is/is not a cause/consequence of X?
- What is the main cause/consequence of X?
- What does X achieve/aim to achieve?
- X is/causes Y because …

Strategy: Always remember and apply the following definitions.

1. Cause: something happens as a direct result of this
2. Consequence: something that happens as a direct result of a cause
3. Bridging phrases: establishes causality e.g. 'because'; 'as a result' etc.

Educated Guessing

There is no negative marking. So, if in doubt, guess!

When guessing, go with your gut instinct. Your subconscious might have absorbed more than you realise. That niggling feeling in the back of your mind is often the result of genuine subconscious analysis.

If you really can't decide which option to go for, then choose 'Can't Tell'. Don't get bogged down on one statement.

> **Top Tip:** If you're stuck, guess and move on. Understanding the clue words can help you to improve your odds by making 'educated guesses'.

Top Verbal Reasoning Tips

- Practice skimming passages for key words/phrases
- Practice reading on a computer screen
- Practice both Question Set formats
- Recognise definitive or mitigating 'clue' words
- Ask why the question writer has put these words in
- Don't get stuck on one question – go with your gut instinct
- Never use outside knowledge
- Never assume causal relationships that aren't stated
- Write your own questions to get in the mindset

Time for some practice! Try answering the following **11 Practice Sets**. Stick to the time limit of **2 minutes per set, and 30 seconds per statement**. Detailed explanations are provided. Good luck!

Practice Sets

Question 1

On October 14, 2012, 43-year-old Austrian Felix Baumgartner floated into space in a capsule suspended from a stratospheric balloon. When the balloon reached 128,000 feet, Felix jumped from the capsule's ledge towards the Earth's surface. The time it took Felix to reach the ground after leaving the capsule was 9 minutes and 3 seconds; 4 minutes and 20 seconds of this time was spent in free fall. Felix reached a maximum velocity of 833.9 mph.

The jump was almost aborted when Felix's helmet visor fogged up during his ascent into space. As he went through last-minute checks inside the capsule, it was found that a heater for his visor was not working. This meant the visor fogged up as he exhaled. 'This is very serious, Joe', he told retired US Air Force Col Joe Kittinger, whose records he was attempting to break, and who was acting as his radio link in mission control at Roswell airport.

Prior to Felix's jump, Kittinger held the records for highest, farthest and longest free fall. These were set when he leapt from a helium envelope in 1960. Felix failed to break Kittinger's record for the longest free fall. After the jump, Felix thanked Kittinger for providing advice and encouragement throughout his preparation and during the jump itself.

1. Felix returned to the Earth's surface 9 minutes and 3 seconds after leaving it in a stratospheric balloon.

    A. True

    B. False

    C. Can't Tell

2. During his 1960 jump, Joe Kittinger was in free fall for more than 4 minutes and 20 seconds.

    A. True

    B. False

    C. Can't Tell

3. Joe Kittinger reassured Felix via radio when his visor fogged up.

    A. True

    B. False

    C. Can't Tell

4. Felix broke the sound barrier during his jump.

    A. True

    B. False

    C. Can't Tell

Question 2

On 29 July 1908, Harland and Wolff presented the drawings for a proposed new ship to the chairman of the White Star Line, J Bruce Ismay. These drawings were approved and work began on a truly vast vessel. The finished ship was 882 feet 9 in long and weighed 46,328 tonnes. Due to its unprecedented size, it was suggested that this ship should be called *Titanic*.

Shortly after 11.40 pm on 14 April 1912, this ship hit an iceberg in the North Atlantic. This created a series of holes below the waterline. The flooding of four of the watertight compartments might have been withstood. Five was too many. The ship sank, bow first, on April 15, 1912. There were only enough lifeboats to accommodate half of the people onboard. Had the ship been carrying its full capacity of 3,339, this would have been reduced to one-third.

The wreck of the ship lies 12,000 feet below the ocean surface. It was found in 1985 by a Franco-American expedition. The team discovered that it had split apart, probably near or at the surface, before sinking to the seabed. Out of the 1,330 passengers and 870 crew who had been onboard, 1,500 died. After a 2004 expedition, photos were released of possible human remains on the ocean floor.

1. The *Titanic* sunk on April 15, 1912.

    A. True

    B. False

    C. Can't Tell

2. 700 people who had been on board the ship survived.

    A. True

    B. False

    C. Can't Tell

3. The ship would not have sunk if only four compartments had flooded.

    A. True

    B. False

    C. Can't Tell

4. There were enough lifeboats to accommodate half the ship's capacity.

    A. True

    B. False

    C. Can't Tell

Question 3

Malaria is one of the developing world's big killers. Without a vaccine, efforts to contain the parasite rely on less effective measures to prevent transmission from mosquitoes, such as insecticide spray and bed nets. However, with many malaria-endemic countries, particularly their rural areas which lack these resources, it has been difficult to stop people dying from the disease.

A recent report by the World Health Organisation (WHO) showed that 4.3 million deaths were prevented between 2001 and 2013 – with the majority of these being young children in sub-Saharan Africa. Clearly, programmes implemented to reduce the number of people dying from the illness have paid off: current estimates claim that 50% of those at risk of malaria infection have access to a mosquito-repellent bed net.

In addition to mosquito nets, access to diagnostic testing and treatment has been improved.

The infection is caused by a parasite that is transmitted by mosquitoes. There are several different types of parasite, with *Plasmodium falciparum* – the most prevalent strain in Africa, where 90% of malaria deaths occur – causing the most severe symptoms. Patients usually suffer from high fever, aching muscles, lack of energy, and headache.

In light of the progress made, several countries are now aiming for total malaria elimination. Azerbaijan and Sri Lanka, for example, reported zero indigenous cases in 2013.

However, if the tools we currently use to fight malaria cease to work, the current success rate cannot be maintained. Emerging drug- and insecticide-resistance of mosquitoes poses a significant potential barrier to malaria elimination. The WHO has also warned that the Ebola outbreak of 2014 could trigger new malaria outbreaks in previously well-controlled regions.

Therefore, it is important that funding for reducing malaria infection continues, and that research towards a vaccine continues.

1. Which of the following can be deduced from the passage?

    A. Malaria is the world's biggest killer.

    B. Vaccines are more effective at stopping transmission than bed nets.

    C. Young children are most at risk from malaria.

    D. 90% of *P. falciparum* parasites can be found in Africa.

2. Which of the following is the author most likely to agree with?

    A. More funding is needed to achieve malaria elimination.

    B. Access to diagnostic testing is not as important as access to treatment.

    C. Bed nets and insecticide spray are widely available in rural areas.

    D. Patients with malaria always suffer from a fever.

3. Using the information in the passage, the following statements are definitely true EXCEPT?

    A. Mosquitoes transmit malaria.

    B. More than 2 million deaths in young children have been averted between 2001 and 2013.

    C. Sri Lanka did not report any cases of malaria in 2013.

    D. People suffering in countries affected by Ebola in 2014 may be at an increased risk of malaria infection compared to 2013.

4. Which of the following can be inferred from the passage?

    A. *P. falciparum* is developing resistance to insecticides.

    B. The non-specific, flu-like symptoms caused by malaria means that diagnosis is difficult without the right technology.

    C. Ninety per cent of malaria infections occur in Africa.

    D. Malaria still poses a significant threat to the lives of millions of people.

Question 4

The two highest grossing movies of all time (not taking into account inflation) were both directed by James Cameron. His 2009 movie, *Avatar*, has taken more than any other film in history: $2.8 billion worldwide. Featuring the blue extra-terrestrials of the Na'vi tribe, who live on the habitable moon of Pandora, the 162-minute epic revolutionised the way 3D technology was used. At the centre of the plot is a romance between one of the Na'vi, Neytiri, and a human called Jake Sully. Sully has been sent to Pandora on behalf of a mining expedition to extract the valuable mineral 'unobtainium'. But when he and Neytiri fall in love, he ends up fighting for her tribe against his former employers.

Titanic is director Cameron's next highest grossing film, taking $2.3 billion overall. The movie revolves around a romance between a blue-collar nomad called Jack Dawson and an aristocratic lady, Rose DeWitt Bukater. *Titanic* was first released in 1997. After it was re-released in 3D in April 2012, it took an additional $364 million, which is included in its overall gross takings. The movie was budgeted at $200 million and was the most expensive film ever made when it was released.

When the numbers are adjusted for inflation, the list of highest-grossing films looks different. *Avatar* drops to second place and is trumped by *Gone with the Wind*. Since its release in 1939, the 220-minute epic has taken $3.3 billion. Two films directed by Steven Spielberg enter the list of the top ten highest grossing films when it is adjusted for inflation: *E.T. the Extra-Terrestrial* ($2.2 billion) and *Jaws* ($1.9 billion). *Titanic* falls to number four, as it is overtaken by *Star Wars*.

1. *Avatar* and *Titanic* are the highest-grossing movies of all time (not taking into account inflation).

    A. True

    B. False

    C. Can't Tell

2. Steven Spielberg's two entries on the top ten highest-grossing film list (adjusted for inflation) both feature non-human characters.

    A. True

    B. False

    C. Can't Tell

3. Multiple James Cameron films feature romances between characters from different backgrounds.

    A. True

    B. False

    C. Can't Tell

4. *Titanic* took in more than $2 billion before April 2012.

    A. True

    B. False

    C. Can't Tell

Question 5

The near-extinction of the dinosaurs occurred around 66 million years ago. We should say 'near-extinction', rather than 'extinction', since there are species of birds that are technically dinosaurs and live to this day. The technical name given to this 'near-extinction' is the 'Cretaceous–Paleogene extinction event' – or the 'K-Pg extinction event', for short. It marks the end of the Mesozoic Era and begins the Cenozoic Era. In the 1970s, palaeontologists started to come up with a variety of theories to explain the K-Pg event. There are fundamentally two schools of thought. One says that it was caused by an impact event, such as an asteroid collision. The other suggests that a confluence of various circumstances resulted in dinosaurs vanishing abruptly from the fossil records.

Within the fossil records, the time of the K-Pg extinction is marked by a thin layer of sediment known as the 'K-Pg boundary'. The boundary clay shows high levels of the metal iridium, which is rare in the Earth's crust but abundant in asteroids. This raises the possibility that the K-Pg event was caused by a giant asteroid or comet, which led to disturbances to the environment including the temporary shutdown of photosynthesis by land plants and plankton. The identification of the 110-mile-wide Chicxulub crater in Mexico provided conclusive evidence that the K-Pg boundary clay contained debris from an asteroid impact.

Among the other possible reasons for the K-Pg extinction, some palaeontologists point to climate change caused by decreasing volcanic activity. This would have cooled the Earth significantly. Research proves that prior to the K-Pg extinction event, the Earth's poles had been 50 degrees centigrade hotter than they are today. Other scientists point to evidence of a significant drop in oxygen levels as the cause of the K-Pg extinction event. If large dinosaurs had respiratory systems similar to birds, this may have meant they became unable to fulfil the significant oxygen requirements of their bodies.

1. Which of the following can be logically inferred from the passage?

    A. There are two different theories put forward by palaeontologists to explain the K-Pg extinction event.

    B. Palaeontologists named the near-extinction of the dinosaurs the Cretaceous–Paleogene extinction event.

    C. Palaeontologists did not come up with theories to explain the K-Pg extinction event prior to 1970.

    D. Palaeontologists only became aware of the K-Pg extinction event during the 1970s.

2. Which of the following statements, if true, would be most likely to weaken the argument that the K-Pg extinction event was caused by a comet or asteroid?

    A. The Chicxulub crater was re-measured and found to be only 100 miles wide, rather than 110 miles wide.

    B. High levels of iridium were found in fossil records from after the K-Pg extinction event.

    C. Small traces of iridium were found in fossil records from before the K-Pg extinction event.

    D. The K-Pg boundary is found to relate to a different time period, much later than first thought.

3. The passage best supports which of the following statements?

   A. Climate change can lead to a decrease in volcanic activity.

   B. Large dinosaurs have similar respiratory systems to birds.

   C. The Earth was hotter over 66 million years ago than it is today.

   D. Oxygen levels dropped dramatically before the K-Pg extinction event.

4. If the passage is true, which of the following is also true?

   A. The Cenozoic Era came before the Mesozoic Era.

   B. The Cenozoic Era followed the Mesozoic Era but not directly.

   C. There were no dinosaurs in the Cenozoic.

   D. The Mesozoic Era directly preceded the Cenozoic Era.

Question 6

Seasonal affective disorder (SAD) describes a type of depression that is affected by seasonal changes in weather, usually occurring during winter. Those who suffer from SAD can experience lethargy, very low mood and frequent cravings for sugary snacks. The condition was first described by the psychiatrist Norman Rosenthal in 1984, and it is now widely known in the modern community.

Less well-known, however, is the exact distinction between true SAD and the less pronounced effect of 'winter blues'. General winter blues are evident to all of us living in seasonal climates, but the work of Rosenthal and others established that the darkness and cold affected the mood of some people much more than others. 'It becomes a medical thing when it has consequences in people's lives, like not being able to get to work or their quality of life going down the drain,' said Rosenthal.

Winter blues often cause difficulty sleeping, while people who suffer from SAD are constantly tired and spend longer resting. Experts claim that between 3% and 5% of the UK population might have SAD, with 12.5% having the more mundane winter blues – a much less well-defined change in mood.

To treat SAD, Rosenthal advocated exposure to special electric lights to counteract the effects of winter darkness and cold. This method of 'light therapy' is actually long established, with Hippocrates documenting the health benefits of sun exposure during the Age of Pericles, and more current evidence also showing light therapy to be successful in improving mood and minimizing SAD symptoms. Despite this, in 2009 the National Institute for Health and Care Excellence (NICE) disappointingly said that there was not enough evidence to justify the NHS covering the cost of light therapy to treat depression.

For now, therefore, SAD remains a condition that sees almost one in twenty people in the UK severely depressed for a significant part of the year. How this subsequently affects society and the economy is something that remains unknown.

1. Which of the following is mainly addressed by the passage?

   A. Why some people are affected by 'winter blues' and others by SAD.

   B. The difference between SAD and 'winter blues'.

C. The scientific basis of light therapy.

D. Rosenthal's career.

2. The author suggests which of the following outcomes?

   A. Patients suffering from SAD are going to be well-cared for in the future.

   B. The prevalence of SAD is on the rise in the UK.

   C. Treatment for SAD is gaining recognition.

   D. SAD may be significantly affecting the UK's society and economy.

3. According to the passage, the author would agree with which of the following statements:

   A. Winter blues and SAD are both medical disorders.

   B. Light therapy is an effective treatment.

   C. Hippocrates suffered from SAD.

   D. All patients suffering from SAD crave sugary snacks.

4. Which of the following questions is NOT answered in the passage?

   A. How common is SAD in the UK population?

   B. When did Rosenthal first describe SAD?

   C. Are there treatments available other than light therapy?

   D. Is light therapy available free of charge?

Question 7

The construction of the Eiffel Tower finished in 1889, and it served as the entrance to that year's World's Fair. It was, in 1889, the tallest building in the world, and remained so until the opening of the Chrysler Building in New York, 41 years later. The Eiffel Tower stands at 1,050 feet high (including an antenna that was added in 1957).

Work on the foundations of the Eiffel Tower started in January 1887. The actual iron work commenced after these were finished in June of that year. The 18,000 parts needed to construct the Eiffel Tower were detailed in 3,000 plan drawings. Many of the parts were riveted together in a factory in the Parisian suburb of Levallois-Perret, and were taken to the site by horse and cart. The Eiffel Tower is made of iron. Obviously, iron rusts unless it is treated with chemicals which can be found in certain types of paint. The Eiffel Tower is coated with 50–60 tonnes of paint every 7 years. Three different colours are typically used, to enhance the lighting effects on the tower.

In its long history, the Eiffel Tower has seen many interesting events and landmarks. Soon after its opening, in September 1889, it was visited by Thomas Edison, who signed the guestbook. Upon the German occupation of Paris in 1940, the lift cables of the Tower were cut by the French so that Adolf Hitler would have to climb the steps. It was said that Hitler conquered France, but did not conquer the Eiffel Tower. On November 28, 2002, the Eiffel Tower received its 200 millionth guest.

1. The 1,050 foot Eiffel Tower was the world's tallest building in 1889.

   A. True

   B. False

   C. Can't Tell

2. Thomas Edison and Adolf Hitler have visited the Eiffel Tower.

   A. True

   B. False

   C. Can't Tell

3. Each plan drawing detailed six of the Eiffel Tower's parts.

   A. True

   B. False

   C. Can't Tell

4. The Eiffel Tower is painted every 7 years to prevent rust.

   A. True

   B. False

   C. Can't Tell

Question 8

New space exploration of Mars has discovered more convincing evidence than ever before of the previous presence of water on the planet. The National Aeronautics and Space Administration (NASA) scientists believe that a large mountain situated at the landing site of their robot, *Curiosity*, was created by layers of sediment being laid down by lakes over millions of years. This hypothesis suggests that the Red Planet is far warmer and wetter than initially thought.

Mount Sharp, the mountain that exists today, stands 5000 metres in height and is believed to have formed when forceful winds and storms eroded the surrounding rock over time.

It is now even thought possible that ancient Mars had snow, rain, and even oceans. These new beliefs build upon previous findings by *Curiosity* on other parts of the planet surface, including banded sediments that followed a pattern suggestive of ancient rivers, deltas and lakes. Uniformly banded patterns of sediment, arranged in a concentric, fluid way around Mount Sharp, gave evidence for the initial connection between sediment deposition and mountain formation.

Through these new discoveries, scientists are recognizing the true value of land exploration, as opposed to only satellite imaging of the surface of Mars, which were not detailed enough to identify Mount Sharp.

Many unanswered questions still remain, and the *Curiosity* team now needs to estimate a time frame for the flow of these rivers and lakes. In addition, existing climate models indicate Mars experienced temperatures far too low to allow water to flow freely. The unique greenhouse effect here on planet Earth, climate experts argue, is a remarkable phenomenon that allows much higher temperatures to be achieved compared to other planets, including Mars. Assessing the time span of the creation of Mount Sharp would allow further understanding of climate evolution on Mars to be developed.

1. Which of the following provides the best summary of the passage?

   A. The use of robots to explore space.

   B. How the greenhouse effect allows for warm temperatures on the Earth.

C. New evidence for the presence of water on Mars.

D. The formation of rivers and deltas.

2. The author would agree with which of the following statements:

A. Evidence for water having existed on Mars is undisputed.

B. There is increasing evidence for water having existed on Mars.

C. The formation of Mount Sharp took place over hundreds of thousands of years.

D. Patterns of sedimentation deposition are definitive evidence of the presence of water.

3. Which of the following questions is NOT answered in the passage?

A. Which space company conducted the *Curiosity* mission?

B. Could Mount Sharp have been explored using satellite imaging?

C. Was there a greenhouse effect on Mars?

D. Why is Mars called the Red Planet?

4. The author suggests which of the following as the key area of further research?

A. The greenhouse effect.

B. Formation of rivers and deltas.

C. Timeframe of Mount Sharp's formation.

D. Improvement of satellite imaging.

Question 9

In 2011, a new single fossil was discovered that confirmed prior belief that *Australopithecus afarensis* – the human ancestor made famous by the Lucy skeleton – mobilized fully upright. In comparison to the same bone in a modern-day human foot, it shares the same features that allow bipedal locomotion.

Unearthed at a known *A. afarensis* fossil site in Ethiopia, the 3.2-million-year-old fossil is one of five long bones that connect the back of the foot to the toes. The fossil's size and shape allowed scientists to determine that the foot it belonged to was stiff and had a well-defined arch – two features that help modern humans spring forward on two feet and that cushion the shock of bipedal walking.

Scientists had already known from pelvis fossils that *A. afarensis* could walk on two legs and no longer had the apelike 'foot thumbs' used by other human ancestral species for grasping and climbing. Before the discovery of the new *A. afarensis* metatarsal, though, it had been hard to say for sure whether Lucy and her kin had left the trees for good.

The fossil gave many more important clues about the way *A. afarensis* lived. For instance, the disappearance of the grasping toe, used in climbing by ape-like species, in favour of the bones of a modern foot, tells us that being mobile on the ground was vital for survival and reproduction. Efficient bipedal walking would have allowed *A. afarensis* to leave forests entirely to search for food or to colonize other areas, for example.

1. Which of the following can be deduced from the passage?

    A. A. afarensis was more ape than human.

    B. Efficient bipedal walking was necessary to find materials to make tools.

    C. A well-defined arch in the foot facilitates bipedal walking.

    D. A. afarensis still lived predominantly in forests.

2. Which of the following is the author most likely to agree with?

    A. Much information about the way a species lived can be deduced from fossil findings.

    B. Pelvis fossils were not informative.

    C. The earliest human fossils were found in Ethiopia.

    D. More funding is needed to help discover new fossils that will tell us more about A. afarensis.

3. Using the information in the passage, the following statements are true EXCEPT?

    A. Bipedal locomotion was vital for efficient mobilization on the ground.

    B. Several A. afarensis skeletons have been discovered.

    C. Humans have five metatarsals in each foot.

    D. A. afarensis was the same standing height as a modern human.

4. Which of the following questions is NOT answered in the passage?

    A. How old is the fossil?

    B. Was the fossil part of a complete skeleton?

    C. How old is Lucy the skeleton?

    D. What was the 'foot thumb' used for?

Question 10

Robert Mugabe has been the leader of Zimbabwe for the three decades of its independence. He was a key figure in the struggle for independence, which involved a bitter bush war against a white minority which had cut the country loose from the colonial power Britain.

When he was first elected in 1980 he was praised for reaching out to the white minority and his political rivals, as well as for what was considered a pragmatic approach to the economy. However, he was soon expelled from the Government of National Unity, the party whose strong-hold was in the south of the country, and launched an anti-opposition campaign in which thousands died.

In the mid-1990s Mugabe embarked on a programme of land redistribution, in which commercial farmers were driven off the land by mobs. The programme was accompanied by a steady decline in the economy. As the opposition to his rule increased, he and his ruling Zanu-PF party grew more determined to stay in power. Critics accuse him of heading a military regime.

In the elections of 2008, Zanu-PF lost its parliamentary majority and opposition leader Morgan Tsvangirai defeated Mr Mugabe in the presidential vote, but with insufficient votes to avoid a run-off. Mr Mugabe was sworn in for another term in June 2008 after a widely condemned run-off vote from which Mr Tsvangirai withdrew because of physical attacks on his supporters. Because of international pressure, Mr Mugabe agreed a power-sharing deal with Mr Tsvangirai, who was made prime minister. (Adapted from http://www.bbc.co.uk/news/world-africa-14113249)

1. Mugabe's land redistribution programme:

    A. Caused a negative impact on Zimbabwe's economy

    B. Took place in the early 1990s

    C. Saw armed mobs drive commercial farmers off land

    D. Coincided with an economic downturn

2. Which of the following was not a consequence of the 2008 elections?

    A. Attacks on Mr Tsvangirai's supporters

    B. Mugabe was made prime minister

    C. A run-off took place

    D. Mugabe was sworn in for another term

3. Mugabe's approach to the economy:

    A. Was based on a programme of land distribution

    B. Was positively received at first

    C. Caused a steady decline

    D. Was likened by critics to that of a military regime

4. Which of the following can be inferred from the passage?

    A. Mugabe did not have much support in south Zimbabwe.

    B. Mugabe used violence to hold on to power.

    C. Mugabe is susceptible to international pressure.

    D. Mugabe was the main figure in Zimbabwe gaining independence.

Question 11

We all know how tempting it can be to have one too many chocolates or an extra slice of cake, even when we know it would be healthier not to. But what drives this craving for sweet treats? Many scientists suggest that we are primed to desire sugar at an instinctive level as it plays such a vital role in our survival. Our sense of taste has evolved to covet the molecules vital to life like salt, fat and sugar.

When we eat food, the simple sugar glucose is absorbed from the intestines into the bloodstream and distributed to all cells of the body. Glucose is particularly important to the brain as it provides a major source of fuel to the billions of neuronal nerve cells. Neurons need a constant supply from the bloodstream as they don't have the ability to store glucose themselves. As diabetics know, someone with low blood sugar can quickly lapse into a coma.

According to the NHS, added sugars shouldn't make up more than 10% of the energy you get from food and drink each day. This is whether it comes from honey, fruit juice and jam, or soft drinks, processed foods or table sugar. This works out at about 70 g a day for men and 50 g for women, although this can vary depending on your size, age and how active you are. Fifty grams of sugar is equivalent to 13 teaspoons of sugar a day, or two cans of fizzy drink, or eight chocolate biscuits.

When in the supermarket it's worth remembering that produce is classed as high in sugar if it contains more than 15 g in 100 g and low in sugar if it has less than 5 g per 100 g. (Adapted from http://www.bbc.co.uk/science/0/21835302)

1. Which of the following statements is best supported by the passage?

   A. We are primed to desire sugar at an instinctive level.

   B. Added sugars shouldn't make up more than 10% of your daily energy.

   C. Low blood sugar levels can lead to a coma.

   D. All men should limit their added sugar intake to 70 g of sugar per day.

2. Which of the following is not true?

   A. Glucose fuels neuronal nerve cells.

   B. 50 g of sugar is equivalent to 13 teaspoons, two fizzy drinks and eight chocolate biscuits.

   C. Produce with more than 15 g in 100 g is classed as high sugar in supermarkets.

   D. Neurons can't store glucose.

3. 50 g of added sugar:

   A. Is the recommended daily intake, according to the NHS

   B. Is the ideal daily amount for every woman

   C. Is found in two fizzy drinks

   D. Is found in eight chocolate biscuits

4. Which of the following can be a consequence of low blood sugar?

   A. Diabetes

   B. Sudden coma

   C. Fainting

   D. Death

Answers

Question 1

1. False

    We know from the first paragraph that it took Felix 9 minutes and 3 seconds to reach the Earth 'after leaving the capsule'. However, we also know that he floated to 128,000 feet, suspended from a stratospheric balloon, before jumping from the capsule ledge. We can safely assume that this took some time. The answer, therefore, is 'False'.

2. True

    The key words are 'free fall'. We know from the first paragraph that Felix spent 4 minutes and 20 seconds in free fall. We know from the third paragraph that Joe Kittinger set the record for the longest free fall during his jump in 1960, and that Felix did not break this record. We can therefore infer that Kittinger was in free fall for longer than 4 minutes and 20 seconds.

3. Can't Tell

    We know from the second paragraph that Felix's visor fogged up. We know that he communicated this to Kittinger via radio. However, even though Felix did eventually jump, the passage does not say anywhere that Kittinger gave him any reassurance on this particular matter. Though the last paragraph refers to general 'advice and encouragement' given to Felix by Kittinger, this does not mean he reassured him about his visor fogging up.

4. Can't Tell

    We know that Felix reached a 'maximum velocity of 833.9 mph'. However, the passage does not give the sound of speed. Nor does it state that Felix broke the sound barrier. You might personally know the speed of sound is 761.2 mph. You might also have read in the news that Felix did, famously, break the sound barrier. But it is important that you do not bring outside knowledge into your reasoning. Based only on the information given in the passage, the answer is 'Can't Tell'.

Question 2

1. Can't Tell

    We know from the second paragraph that the ship described sank on April 15, 1912. But the only mention of the name *Titanic* is in the first paragraph: 'it was **suggested** that this ship should be called *Titanic*'. Although outside knowledge might tell us that this name was indeed adopted, using information in the passage alone we only know that the name *Titanic* was suggested. We do not know if this was the name that was actually given to the ship. Therefore, the answer is 'Can't Tell'.

2. True

    The last paragraph says: 'out of the 1,330 passengers and 870 crew onboard, 1,500 died'. We know from this that there were 1,330 + 870 = 2,200 people onboard. If 1,500 died, then 2,200 – 1,500 = 700 survived.

3. Can't Tell

The key word is 'compartments'. Paragraph two says: 'four of the watertight compartments flooding might have been withstood'. The word 'might' tells us that we do not know for sure whether four compartments flooding would have sunk the ship. Therefore, the answer is 'Can't Tell'.

4. False

From the end of the second paragraph, we know that: 'there were only enough lifeboats to accommodate half of the people *onboard*.' But we are interested in how many of its *capacity* the lifeboats could accommodate. The next sentence says: 'had the ship been carrying its full capacity of 3,339, this would have been reduced to one third.' Therefore, there were only enough lifeboats to carry one third, rather than one half, of the ship's capacity.

Question 3

1. B

The answer to this question can be located in the passage by scanning for key words and then reading the full sentence, as well as those before and after. In linking the words 'without' [a vaccine] and 'rely on less effective measures' [bed nets], we can infer from the passage that vaccines are superior to bed nets at stopping 'people dying from the disease' (in the sentence after the key word).

2. A

Questions that ask you to judge what the author is 'most likely' to agree with will usually require you to read the passage in full to gain an overall understanding of the author's message. In this instance, however, the answer can be pinpointed by scanning for the word 'funding' – the key word in the first answer. Nevertheless, you should make sure to quickly scan for the other potential answers as well, to ensure you do not jump to conclusions.

3. C

Although 'zero' may seem to be a Definitive Word, the passage states that there were 'zero indigenous cases' – in other words, cases may have been present in Sri Lanka, even though they were brought into the country by travellers, rather than occurring in the local population. While Option C therefore initially looks to be true, the evidence we are given is not definitive. Option A is stated in the first paragraph about prevention, while Option B is definitely true because the passage claims the 'majority' of the 4.3 million deaths averted to have been in young children: 2 million is less than half of this figure. Finally, the use of the same Mitigating Word ('may') in the question and answer ('may be at increased risk', and 'may trigger new malaria outbreaks') means in this case that Option D is definitely true.

4. D

Questions about what can be inferred from the passage are among the hardest type. They require you not only to understand the overall message of the author, but also put your feet in his shoes, and judge what he or she would think of the statements ... all within the context of what was discussed in the passage! Options B and C here try to trick you into employing Outside Knowledge, while Option A is Faulty Logic: although the passage states that mosquitoes are developing resistance and that *P. faliciparum* is a mosquito, we cannot necessarily infer that *P. faliciparum* is developing resistance. Option A is therefore correct – and this is an overall message that is reiterated throughout the passage.

Question 4

1. True

    Looking for the first key words – 'highest-grossing movies of all time (not taking into account inflation)' – leads us straight to the first line, where we read that the top two were both directed by James Cameron. The next sentence gives more relevant information, saying that 'his' film, '*Avatar*', our next key word, 'has taken more than any other film in history'. This is the same as saying that it is the highest grossing film of all time (before inflation). Our next key word is '*Titanic*', and we first see this at the start of the second paragraph, where we are told it is: 'Cameron's next highest grossing film, taking $2.3 billion'. Since we know that Cameron directed the two highest grossing films of all time, and we know that Avatar was the highest grossing film of all time, we can infer that if *Titanic* was *Cameron's* second-highest grossing film, it was also *the* second-highest grossing film of all time. So the answer is 'True'.

2. Can't Tell

    Searching for mention of 'Spielberg' takes us to the end of the third paragraph. We can verify from this that: 'two films directed by Steven Spielberg enter the top ten highest grossing films list when it is adjusted for inflation'. We are also told that these are titled *E.T. the Extra-Terrestrial* and *Jaws*. However, we are told nothing in the passage about the content of these films, so we have no idea if they feature 'non-human characters'. Remember not to bring in outside knowledge! It is also not true to say that the film title *E.T. the Extra-Terrestrial* logically infers the presence of a 'non-human character' since film titles are not necessarily descriptive. (For example, *Reservoir Dogs* contains neither dogs nor a reservoir.) Even if it did, however, *Jaws* could refer to anything in this context.

3. True

    We need to look for the key word 'romance'. In the first paragraph, this will tell us that in Cameron's *Avatar* 'the centre of the plot is a romance between one of the Na'vi, Neytiri, and a human called Jake Sully'. This certainly classifies as a romance between characters from different backgrounds. But in order to verify the statement, we need to know if this is the case in 'multiple' Cameron films, i.e. *more* than one. Continuing to look for the key word 'romance' we get to the second paragraph. Here we are told that Cameron's *Titanic* 'revolves around a romance between a blue-collar nomad called Jack Dawson and an aristocratic lady, Rose DeWitt Bukater'. This also fits the description of a romance between characters from different backgrounds. The answer is therefore 'True'.

4. False

    We are looking for figures relating to *Titanic*. This takes us only to the second paragraph. We know from the first sentence that the movie took $2.3 billion. But if we look for the key words 'April 2012', we learn that this number includes $364 million taken *after* the film was re-released in 3D on that date. Since $2.3 billion minus $364 million is less than $2 billion, the film cannot have taken more than $2 billion *before* that date. The answer is therefore 'False'.

Question 5

1. C

   Locating the keyword '1970s' leads us to the line: 'In the 1970s, palaeontologists started to come up with a variety of theories to explain the K-Pg extinction event'. The word 'started' logically infers that this had not happened before the 1970s, which began in 1970. None of the other statements can be logically inferred from the passage:

   A. Though we are told that there are 'fundamentally two schools of thought', in this context 'fundamentally' acts as a mitigating term, meaning 'broadly speaking' or 'for the most part'. The preceding sentence also tells us explicitly that there are 'a variety of theories'. Some of these are even highlighted in the final paragraph.

   B. Though we are told that Cretaceous–Paleogene extinction event was 'the technical name given' to the near extinction of the dinosaurs, we do not know if it was given by palaeontologists.

   D. We know that palaeontologists 'started to come up with a variety of theories' to explain the K-Pg event in the 1970s, but this is not the same as saying they only became aware of it in the 1970s.

2. D

   In order to get the answer we need to go through each statement, one by one. Our thought process for each statement should work as follows:

   A. This is a clear decoy. There is no evidence that altering the measurement of the Chicxulub crater by less than 10% would have any impact on the asteroid/comet theory.

   B. This might suggest another asteroid after the K-Pg extinction event, but this would not make it less likely that one caused the K-Pg extinction event in the first place.

   C. 'Small traces' of iridium is consistent with the fact that the passage tells us that iridium is 'rare' in the Earth's crust. Had there been high levels of iridium prior to the K-Pg extinction event, we might have inferred that there was another asteroid prior to the K-Pg extinction event that the dinosaurs survived, which could have weakened the argument.

   D. The theory of the asteroid or comet causing the K-Pg extinction event is heavily reliant on the high levels of iridium found in the K-Pg boundary. If this layer of sediment in fact related to a later time period, significantly after the K-Pg extinction event, this would therefore significantly weaken the argument.

3. C

   In order to get the answer we need to go through each statement, one by one. Our thought process for each statement should work as follows:

   A. Reference to climate change and volcanic activity leads us to the start of the final paragraph, where we are told that some people cite 'climate change caused by decreasing volcanic activity' as a reason for the K-Pg extinction event. This is, in fact, directly opposed to the statement, which suggests it is climate change that can lead to a decrease in volcanic activity, rather than vice versa.

B. Looking for key terms takes us to the last sentence, where we are told that 'if large dinosaurs had respiratory systems similar to birds' it might support theories about a drop in oxygen levels leading to the K-Pg extinction event. 'If' is a clear mitigation and suggests the statement is speculative – we do not know if large dinosaurs did in fact have respiratory systems similar to birds.

C. The information in this statement is split across the passage. Reference to '66 million years ago' takes us to the first paragraph, where we learn that this was approximately when the K-Pg extinction event occurred. Reference to the temperature of the Earth leads us to the final paragraph, where we are told that before the K-Pg extinction event, 'the Earth's poles had been 50 degrees centigrade hotter than they are today.' Linking these two pieces of information means that the passage therefore supports the assertion that the Earth was hotter over 66 million years ago than it is today.

D. Should we need to check the final statement, we would learn from the passage that 'some scientists point to evidence of a significant drop in oxygen levels'. The fact that there is evidence of a significant drop in oxygen levels, and that some scientists point to this, is not the same as saying there *was* a significant drop in oxygen levels. So while this could be true, it is less likely than option C.

4. D

The words 'Mesozoic' and 'Cenozoic' occur in the first paragraph, where we are told that the K-Pg extinction event 'marks the end of the Mesozoic Era and begins the Cenozoic Era'. Since the word 'preceded' means 'comes before', this confirms that the Mesozoic Era 'preceded' the Cenozoic Era. And since the same event marked the end of the Mesozoic and the start of the Cenozoic Era, we can also verify that it preceded it 'directly'. The other statements are all false or uncertain:

A. For the reasons above, we know that the Mesozoic Era came before the Cenozoic Era, rather than vice versa.

B. It is true that the Cenozoic Era followed the Mesozoic Era, but for the reasons above we know that it did follow directly.

C. Though the Cenozoic Era followed the K-Pg extinction event, we know that this marked the 'near extinction', rather than the full extinction, of the dinosaurs.

Question 6

1. B

When being asked the 'overall message' or 'main theme' of a piece of text, try to count the frequency at which key topics and their synonyms are mentioned in the paragraph. This will give a rough guide from which to then use your logical assessment of the passage to identify the overall topic of the piece. In this case, 'light therapy' is only mentioned in one section, while Rosenthal's career and the causation of SAD and winter blues are hardly mentioned. The overriding theme is clearly the controversy between the definition of SAD and winter blues.

2. D

The clue to this question is in the final sentence, so make sure your reading is thorough and complete! 'Society' and 'economy' are key words that point you in the direction of the answer, while the Mitigating Word 'may' in the answer allows you to link it to the statement 'effect ... remains unknown' – in other words, highlighting a grey area.

3. B

The passage juxtaposes the 'disappointing' NICE Guidelines with age-old practices of Hippocrates as well as 'up-to-date evidence' to imply that NICE failing to recognize light therapy as an effective treatment is a mistake. It is very likely that the author would there-fore agree that light therapy is a successful treatment option. You can also achieve the same answer by eliminating the other options. Option D uses a Definitive Word ('all') that makes it very unlikely to be correct. Option A is exactly the opposite of what the author is suggesting, while Option B is not stated in the passage and is therefore unknown.

4. C

In many ways, these questions are the easiest to answer. Simply ask yourself to search for the answer in the passage – being careful not to employ Outside Knowledge or Faulty Logic to create answers. In this case, although the author states that NICE currently does not endorse light therapy, no explanations of alternative therapies offered by NICE are outlined in the passage and therefore this is the correct answer.

Question 7

1. False

We can verify in the first paragraph that the Eiffel Tower 'was, in 1889, the tallest build-ing in the world'. Scanning for the given measurement, we can also see that it stands at 1,050 feet high. However, we are also told, in the parentheses, that this measurement is 'including an antenna that was added in 1957'. We can therefore infer that before 1957, the Eiffel Tower was less than 1,050 feet tall. So while it was the world's tallest building in 1889, it was not then 1,050 feet tall. The answer is therefore 'False'.

2. Can't Tell

The key reference points are 'Thomas Edison' and 'Adolf Hitler', both mentioned in the final paragraph. We are told categorically that 'in September 1889, [the Eiffel Tower] was visited by Thomas Edison'. So that part of the statement is verified. In terms of Hitler, we can read that: 'the lift cables of the Tower were cut by the French so that Adolf Hitler would have to climb the steps'. However, this refers to a hypothetical situation – if Hitler visited. There is nothing to tell us whether he actually did or didn't. The phrase: 'It was said that Hitler conquered France, but did not conquer the Eiffel Tower', sheds no further light on this matter. And thus we 'Can't Tell'.

3. Can't Tell

We should scan the passage for the term 'plan drawing', and in particular the numbers of parts included in each of these. In the second paragraph, one sentence tells us that: 'The 18,000 parts needed to construct the Eiffel Tower were detailed in 3,000 plan draw-ings'. If each plan drawing detailed an equal number of parts, we could infer that each one detailed six parts. Since this is not stated or inferred, however, we cannot make this assumption. However, the possibility is not discounted, either. So the answer is 'Can't Tell'.

4. Can't Tell

We know from the end of the second paragraph, having looked for our key phrases, that: 'the Eiffel Tower is coated with 50–60 tonnes of paint every 7 years'. Looking for reference to 'rust' takes us to the preceding sentence, where we are told that: 'iron rusts unless it is treated with chemicals which can be found in certain types of paint'. So the passage confirms two things: (1) the Eiffel Tower is painted every 7 years, and (2) some paints contain anti-rust chemicals. But the passage does not logically infer that the paint used on the Eiffel Tower is in fact the type that does contain anti-rust chemicals, or that the purpose of the 7 yearly painting is to prevent rust. The statements are juxtaposed, but not necessarily directly related, unless by assumption, which is to be avoided. So the answer is 'Can't Tell'.

Question 8

1. C

   By scanning for key words, it is easy to see what the overall meaning of the passage is according to the number of times these words (and their synonyms) occur in the passage. In this case, the word 'water' and the related words of 'flow', 'river', 'lakes', 'fluid' and 'wetter' all suggest that the overall meaning of the passage is related to water. In addition, from reading the information, 'new evidence' is also frequently discussed.

2. B

   Words and phrases such as 'new' and 'even thought' show that the evidence being discussed is building on previous findings: in other words, 'increasing'. The passage states that NASA scientists 'believe' their findings to be true: a Mitigating Word that implies that the presence of water on Mars is not a fact. When being asked about a quantity, scan the passage for any numerical values (including those written in words). This allows you to easily identify that Mount Sharp was formed over millions – not hundreds of thousands – of years.

3. D

   In many ways, these questions are the easiest to answer. Simply ask yourself to search for the answer in the passage, being careful not to employ Outside Knowledge or Faulty Logic to create answers. In this case, there is no mention of 'Red Planet' in the passage, therefore Option D is correct. Make sure, however, to eliminate the other options before committing to an answer. For example, the possessive pronoun 'their' in the first paragraph gives evidence that the *Curiosity* mission was conducted by NASA, so Option A is not the correct answer. The passage also clearly states that satellite imaging lacked the level of detail required to explore Mount Sharp, and that the greenhouse effect is unique to planet Earth – thus answering the questions posed in Options B and C.

4. C

   The word 'further' in the question is key to your targeted reading: you should look towards the end of the passage for the author's suggestions of future implications of the topic being discussed. In this case, use of the key phrase 'time span' in the final sentence of the text gives you the correct answer: to investigate the time course over which Mount Sharp was formed. While the other topics are discussed in the passage, the author does not say anything to imply the need for future research in these areas.

Question 9

1. C

   This question can be easily answered by targeted reading. In the second paragraph, the key words 'bipedal walking' and 'well-defined arch' are used in the same sentence. Remember, again, to quickly assess the validity of the other answers as well.

2. A

   Although this answer can be deduced by the overall theme of the passage, the first sentence of the last paragraph includes the crucial phrase 'many more important clues'. While this is not a factual statement, the question is asking you to assess the author's opinion, and it is clear that he or she strongly believes that much information can be gained from fossil findings. Option C employs Outside Information, while Option B simply contradicts the passage, and Option D is not mentioned by the passage but is therefore susceptible to being chosen as a result of Faulty Logic.

3. D

   This question requires you to scan for key words and their synonyms to choose by exclusion. 'Standing height' is not strictly mentioned, although 'standing' in general is. Therefore Option D is not a true statement based on the passage. Option C is more difficult to exclude: it requires knowledge that 'metatarsals' are bones. However, if you scan for the word 'five', you can deduce this from the context of the passage – which discusses anatomy of the fossils – that the author is discussing bone structure.

4. C

   In many ways, these questions are the easiest to answer. Simply ask yourself to search for the answer in the passage, being careful not to employ Outside Knowledge or Faulty Logic to create answers. In this case, it may be tempting to assume that the passage is describing Lucy the fossil. However, in the first paragraph it is made clear that the topic of discussion is a fossil of the same species as Lucy – thus, the age of Lucy's fossil is not stated in the passage.

Question 10

1. D

   We are told in the third paragraph that 'The [land redistribution] programme was accompanied by a steady decline in the economy'. 'Accompanied' can mean 'happened at the same time as', and a 'steady decline in the economy' fits with 'economic downturn'. Therefore, it is accurate to say that the programme 'coincided with an economic downturn'.

   A. Though we know that the programme was 'accompanied by economic decline', we do not know that the programme was the cause of that decline. Be careful not to assume cause and effect!

   B. The passage clearly says that the programme took place in the mid, rather than 'early', 1990s.

   C. We know that 'mobs' drove commercial farmers off the land. However, there is no evidence that these mobs were 'armed'.

2. B

The final paragraph says that 'Mr Tsvangirai was made prime minister' as part of a power sharing regime. Though Mugabe was earlier 'sworn in', we do not know in what capacity.

A. The previous sentence says that Mr Tsvangirai withdrew from the run-off because of attacks on his supporters.

C. There are two references to this run-off in the final paragraph.

D. As per B, we are told that 'Mugabe was sworn in for another term'.

3. B

The second paragraph says of Mugabe: 'When he was first elected in 1980 he was praised for reaching out to the white minority and his political rivals, *as well as for what was considered a pragmatic approach to the economy*'. Since he was praised for his pragmatic approach to the economy, and this praise came when he was first elected, we can fairly conclude that his economic approach was received positively at first.

A. Though we know this programme was implemented in the mid-1990s, there is no evidence that it was what Mugabe's economic approach was 'based on'.

C. We know there was a 'steady decline in the economy' but we cannot automatically conclude that this was a result of Mugabe's economic approach, since this is not stated. Economic decline can have a number of causes not related to the government's economic approach, e.g. natural disaster.

D. Though critics did liken Mugabe's to a 'military regime', nowhere was this linked to economic policy.

4. C

In the final paragraph, we are told that 'Because of international pressure, Mr Mugabe agreed a power-sharing deal with Mr Tsvangirai, who was made prime minister.' So, we know that there was international pressure, and we know that Mugabe acted 'because of this' – 'because of' being the key bridging phrase.

A. Though we know from the second paragraph that 'he was soon expelled from the Government of National Unity, the party whose stronghold was in the south', this is not the same as saying Mugabe lacked support in the south.

B. There is nothing specifically stating this. Though there is some reference to violence, and a clear reference to the fact that 'he and his ruling Zanu-PF party grew more determined to stay in power', the two things are never explicitly linked with a clear bridging phrase.

D. We know from the first paragraph that Mugabe was 'a key figure in the struggle for independence'. However, being 'a' key figure implies there were others, so saying he was '*the*' key figure is not accurate based on the information given.

Question 11

1. C

The end of the second paragraph says: 'As diabetics know, someone with low blood sugar can quickly lapse into a coma'. The use of the word 'know' is key as it supports the fact that what follows is factually correct. And indeed, the information about people with low blood sugar potentially lapsing into comas is presented in definitive terms – unlike any of the other answer options.

A. We are told in the first paragraph that 'Many scientists suggest' this is the case. That does not mean that it definitely is the case. Since it is less definitive than option C, it is not, therefore, the best supported statement.

B. The third paragraph effectively says this, but the information is introduced with the caveat: 'According to the NHS'. Again, this means it is subjective rather than objective, unlike option C.

D. Again, this follows from the NHS opinion and is therefore subjective. Furthermore, the amount of added sugar will 'vary depending on your size, age and how active you are'. So 70 g will not be an accurate figure for 'all men'.

2. B

This statement is false because of one word: 'and'. The passage says, at the end of the penultimate paragraph, that 50 g of sugar is equivalent to: '13 teaspoons of sugar a day, *or* two cans of fizzy drink, *or* eight chocolate biscuits'. It is possible to miss this detail when scanning quickly, so make sure you hone in on relevant parts of the passage and pick up the requisite level of detail.

A. The second paragraph confirms that glucose is 'a major source of fuel to the billions of neuronal nerve cells'.

C. The final sentence confirms that 'produce is classed as high in sugar if it contains more than 15 g in 100 g'.

D. The second paragraph confirms that 'Neurons need a constant supply from the bloodstream as they don't have the ability to store glucose themselves'.

3. D

The last sentence of the third paragraph says that '[F]ifty grams of sugar is equivalent to … eight chocolate biscuits'. 'Equivalent to' in this context – i.e. referring to sugar content – means that 50 g of sugar is found in eight chocolate biscuits. The full statement – '50 g of sugar is found in eight chocolate biscuits' – would therefore be 'True'.

A. The third paragraph gives 50 g as the daily recommended intake specifically for women. The recommended daily intake for men is 70 g. Therefore, this is an over-generalisation and consequently 'False'.

B. Once again, we must take note of the fact that, though the recommended daily amount for women is 50 g per day, this will 'vary depending on your size, age and how active you are'. So 50 g cannot logically be said to be ideal for *every* woman.

C. By the same logic that makes 'D' the correct answer, we know that 50 g of sugar is found in 'two cans of fizzy drink'. On the face of it, the complete statement – '50 g of sugar is found in two fizzy drinks' – therefore appears to be 'True'. However, the passage specifies that 50 g of sugar is equivalent to two *cans of* fizzy drink. Therefore, the valid response to the full statement would actually be 'Can't Tell' rather than 'True'. If the two fizzy drinks were in cans, then yes, it would be 'True'. But if they were in big, 2-litre bottles, then the answer would be 'False'. We don't know.

4. B

The last sentence of the second paragraph says: 'As diabetics know, someone with low blood sugar can quickly lapse into a coma'. If it had said that 'diabetics think…' or 'diabetics believe…' then we would not be able to tell if what followed was a genuine consequence. However, the verb 'know' is definitive and therefore what follows must be 'True'. The use of the word 'sudden' in the answer is borne out by the use of the word 'quickly' in the passage.

A. There is nothing to support this in the passage alone. Though diabetics know the consequences of low blood sugar, this does not logically affirm that diabetes is a consequence of low blood sugar.

C   There is no mention of this, and this answer would require an assumption.

D. There is no mention of this, and this answer would require an assumption.

CHAPTER 2

Quantitative Reasoning

Overview

The Quantitative Reasoning (QR) Section is the most time pressured part of the UKCAT examination. It challenges students to solve mathematical problems by applying logic and reasoning. Students who aren't studying maths beyond GCSE often feel disadvantaged in this section. But the truth is they aren't! As the UKCAT website says, the QR Section 'assumes familiarity with numbers to the standard of a good pass at GCSE. However items are less to do with numerical facility and more to do with problem solving'. In other words, the emphasis is on logic and reasoning, not complex calculations.

Format of the Section

Students will be presented with nine Scenarios. Each of these Scenarios contains four associated questions. This gives a total of 36 questions. Each question has five answer options. You have 25 minutes in which to complete all 36 questions (including 1 minute of reading time).

Each Scenario begins with a short passage of introductory text. This is followed by some data. The data can be presented in a number of ways, including:

- Tables
- Charts/pie charts
- Graphs
- 2- and 3-Dimensional shapes
- Diagrams
- Pure text with no pictorial representation

Sometimes the answer options include 'Can't Tell'. This means that it is *not possible* to calculate the answer to the question based on the available information. It does not mean that after performing calculations, you disagree with the other answer options. If you think that it is possible to work it out but you have arrived at a different answer, then you've made a mistake.

Mathematical Knowledge

The level of mathematical knowledge required is quite basic. You need to be familiar with:

- Basic arithmetic
- Fractions, decimals and ratios
- Averages
- Percentages
- Common formulas
- Geometrical formulas

The key challenges include correctly identifying which data to use, applying logic and reasoning to solve problems and doing it all under immense time pressure. Even the most basic question can become complicated when you add in the dreaded time factor.

Strategy

This section feels – and is – very time pressured, so it is imperative that you become less reliant on using a calculator by performing mental arithmetic.

You have an average of 40 seconds per question but some questions will take far longer to answer. Strategy, therefore, becomes essential. You need to 'gain time' on easy questions so that you can spend more on the challenging ones.

Whenever looking at a question, you should ask yourself three things:

1. Do I need to do any calculations?

2. Do the numbers work?

3. Can I eliminate any answer options?

Many questions in QR require no calculations at all. They simply involve correctly reading data from the information presented. It seems straightforward. But working under time pressure can make it very challenging in practice!

Students preparing for the QR section often believe they will need to use a calculator for every question. This couldn't be further from the truth. The numbers in QR tend to work quite nicely. They may look complex at first but are often designed in such a way that they can be calculated in your head, or quickly using the booklet provided. There are, of course, questions where you will need to use your calculator. But these are in the minority.

> **Top Tip:** When revising, give yourself six 'tokens' for the QR section. Each time you use a calculator during a full set of 36 QR questions that means you've used one token. This simple rule will help you think twice before using your calculator in future. Eventually, this will make you faster!

You are not allowed to bring a pocket calculator into the exam. You have to use the on-screen one. You can activate this by clicking the 'calculator' button in the top left corner of the screen. The on-screen calculator is very basic, effectively limiting you to addition, subtraction, multiplication and division. There is also a square root button, but that's it. Again, this highlights the fundamental principle of QR: that it has less to do with numbers and more to do with problem solving.

> **Top Tip:** Using the on-screen calculator is significantly more time consuming than using a pocket calculator. So when revising from a textbook, always use your computer's basic calculator (e.g. in the Windows start bar) to answer questions. This allows you to replicate the UKCAT's on-screen calculator, with all the associated difficulties.

Every question in QR has five possible answers. It is, however, usually possible to eliminate one or more options straight away. Some will use the wrong units; others will be in the wrong order of magnitude. So, even if you are tempted to guess on a question, always try to eliminate some implausible options first.

The 'flag' function is particularly important in the QR, because of the intense time pressure. Some questions are more time consuming than others. If you're not vigilant, you may find yourself struggling to finish the section. When you encounter a particularly time-consuming question, your best option is to select a sensible answer (having eliminated obviously incorrect options), before 'flagging' it and moving quickly on.

Remember: Every question is worth one mark. So you're better off finishing the section and answering all the easy one-mark questions than you are answering fewer difficult questions and running out of time. The best 'game strategy', rather than the cleverest answers, will ultimately lead to success.

Common Themes

In the Quantitative Reasoning section there are many common themes, along with subtle tricks to catch you out. The following Example Question Sets will demonstrate how these work in practice. By the end of this section, you will feel much better prepared to tackle the QR section of the UKCAT.

Refer to **Example Set 1**, below. Keep in mind the three golden rules as you work your way through:

1. Do I need to do any calculations?

2. Do the numbers work?

3. Can I eliminate any answers?

Set a timer for 160 seconds and make a note of your answers before moving on to the explanations.

Example Set 1

Motorsport Mania is a racing series where motorsport enthusiasts from around Europe meet once a month to race home built cars. There is one race per month, where the top six drivers score 10, 6, 4, 3, 2 and 1 points, respectively. Each season there are 11 races, with double points being awarded in the final race, which takes place just before Christmas. Following is a table of results for the top 10 drivers:

Position	Driver	Nationality	Points
1	Nathan Fielding	British	92
2	Peter Garside	British	38
3	Kristoffer Bergstrom	Swedish	35
4	Pierre Valerie	French	32
5	Peter Gough	British	20
6	Klaus Spiegelman	German	17
7	Steve Gardiner	Irish	16
8	Fernando Lopez	Spanish	12
9	Paul Johnstone	British	10
10	Marc Alexandre	French	8

1. What is the fewest number of races that the winner of the series could have won?

    A.   2

    B.   3

    C.   4

    D.   5

    E.   Can't Tell

2. On average, how many points did the British drivers score?

    A.   28

    B.   40

    C.   47

    D.   50

    E.   65

3. The winner of each race earns £1000, with a £500 bonus for winning the Christmas race, while the second and third place drivers are only awarded a trophy. There are no other financial prizes awarded. What is the most that the highest scoring French driver could have earned in one season?

    A.   £0

    B.   £2500

    C.   £3000

    D.   £3500

    E.   Can't Tell

4. Nathan Fielding won the final race, completing the race in 120 minutes and 42 seconds. He drove a total distance of 260 kilometres and had two pit stops for fuel, stopping for 19 and 23 seconds each. Excluding his pit stops, what was his average speed?

    A.   129.2 miles per hour

    B.   130 miles per hour

    C.   129.2 kilometres per hour

    D.   130 kilometres per hour

    E.   Can't Tell

Example Set 1: Answers and Explanations

Question 1

What is the fewest number of races that the winner of the series could have won?

ANSWER: D. 5

This question requires you to use some logic when solving the problem. You know that the winner of every race scores 10 points, while the second-placed driver scores 8. You also know that the winner, Nathan Fielding, scored 92 points in total. Assuming that he finished in second place in all races, he would only have scored 72 points. (Remember: the last race scores double points). As such, there is a shortfall of 20 points. The difference between first and second place is 4 points. To make up this shortfall, he would have had to win at least five races (20 divided by 4).

Question 2

On average, how many points did the British drivers score?

ANSWER: B. 40

There are four British drivers, finishing in first, second, fifth and ninth places. Between them they scored a total of 160 points. You should be able to add these values in your head without the need for a calculator. The average number of points scored by British drivers is therefore 160 divided by 4, which equals 40.

Question 3

The winner of each race earns £1000, with a £500 bonus for winning the Christmas race, while the second and third place drivers are only awarded a trophy. There are no other financial prizes awarded. What is the most that the highest scoring French driver could have earned in one season?

ANSWER: C. £3000

The highest scoring French driver is Pierre Valerie, finishing in fourth. He scores a total of 32 points. As the winner of each race scores 10 points he could, at most, have won three races. Therefore he could only have won, at most, 3 x £1000. One of those races could have been the Christmas race, earning him the £500 bonus. But, as he would have earned double points, this means he would only have won one 'normal' race in addition to the Christmas race. The most he could therefore have won in one season is £3000, assuming he won three 'normal' races. Had he won the Christmas race, scoring double points, he could have earned £2500.

Question 4

Nathan Fielding won the final race, completing the race in 120 minutes and 42 seconds. He drove a total distance of 260 kilometres and had two pit stops for fuel, stopping for 19 and 23 seconds each. Excluding his pit stops, what was his average speed?

ANSWER: D. 130 kilometres per hour

This question utilises a favourite formula of the UKCAT:

$$Speed = \frac{Distance}{Time}$$

If you initially asked yourself 'do the numbers work?' then the question would have been straightforward. Although seemingly requiring a calculator, you should quickly be able to see that you need to remove 42 seconds from the original 120 minutes 42 seconds (as Fielding stopped for 19 and 23 seconds), leaving you with 120 minutes, which is equal to 2 hours, at which point the numbers then become easy to work with:

$$Speed = \frac{260}{2} = 130 \; kilometres \; per \; hour$$

When answering the questions, pay close attention to the units. Under time pressure, less than 20% of students answer this question correctly. Many run out of time using a calculator; others select options A and B, which have the wrong units.

For the next questions, please refer to **Example Set 2**. Allow yourself 160 seconds to complete the next four questions, making note of your answers before moving on to the explanations.

Example Set 2

Amanda is having three friends round for dinner, and plans on serving tacos. She requires the following ingredients:

- 600 g extra lean minced meat
- 1 packet of taco shells
- 1 lettuce head
- 1 sachet of taco spice

- 1 jar of salsa

- 1 packet of grated cheese

The distance to Shop 1 is 15 miles, so before leaving she looks online and compares the prices of various ingredients in three shops:

Ingredient	Shop 1	Shop 2	Shop 3
Lettuce (1 head)	£0.80	£0.80	£0.90
Tom's Taco Spice (1 sachet)	£1.25	£1.20	£1.20
300 g minced meat	£4.50	£5.00	£8.85
Taco Shells (1 packet)	£1.50	£1.60	£1.65
Salsa (1 jar)	£1.95	£1.40	£2.25
Cheese (1 packet)	£2.40	£3.00	£3.00

1. If Amanda buys all of her ingredients from Shop 2, what is the cost per person of dinner?

   A. £3.25

   B. £4.50

   C. £6.00

   D. £13.00

   E. £18.00

2. What is the percentage difference in price of a packet of cheese in Shop 3 as compared to Shop 1?

   A. 20%

   B. 25%

   C. 27%

   D. 120%

   E. 125%

3. Amanda buys her ingredients from Shop 3 along with a number of additional items. Her total shopping bill comes to £20.00. How much does the lettuce contribute as a percentage to her total bill?

   A. 4.5%

   B. 5%

   C. 5.75%

   D. 7.2%

   E. 9%

4. The distance to Shop 3 is 20% further than Shop 1, however the route to Shop 3 involves using a motorway, so her average speed travelling to Shop 3, 54 miles per hour, is faster than travelling to Shop 1. How long will it take her to drive to Shop 3?

   A.   20 minutes

   B.   22 minutes

   C.   25 minutes

   D.   27 minutes

   E.   Can't Tell

Example Set 2: Answers and Explanations

Question 1

If Amanda buys all of her ingredients from Shop 2, what is the cost per person of dinner?

ANSWER: B. £4.50

The answer options in the UKCAT are always designed so that each option represents an answer you could have generated if you fell for one of the tricks, and in this question there are several tricks! If you total the price of all items from Shop 2, the total price is £18.00. (Remember: she needs two packets of meat.) However, if you left it at this then you forgot to fully read the question, which asked for the price *per person*. If Amanda has three friends round for dinner, then there are four people in total. The price per person is therefore £4.50.

Question 2

What is the percentage difference in price of a packet of cheese in Shop 3 as compared to Shop 1?

ANSWER: B. 25%

Percentage change is one of the 'must know' formulas for UKCAT:

$$Percentage\ change = \left(\frac{Difference}{Original}\right) \times 100$$

In this scenario, the difference is £0.60 (£3.00 – £2.40) and the original £2.40. The percentage difference is therefore 25%.

Question 3

Amanda buys her ingredients from Shop 3 along with a number of additional items. Her total shopping bill comes to £20.00. How much does the lettuce contribute as a percentage to her total bill?

ANSWER: A. 4.5%

The formula to calculate the percentage that one item accounts for out of the grand total is

$$Percentage = \left(\frac{Given\ amount}{Total\ amount}\right) \times 100$$

As the cost of lettuce is £0.90 and her total shopping bill comes to £20.00, we can calculate that the percentage must be 4.5%.

N.B.: In this scenario, you could have reached the correct answer without the need for any calculations. If you rounded up the price of lettuce to £1, then this would have contributed 5% (1 in 20 = 5%). As the price of lettuce is less than £1, the percentage contribution must have been less than 5%. The only answer option less than 5% is A.

Question 4

The distance to Shop 3 is 20% farther than Shop 1. However, the route to Shop 3 involves using a motorway, so her average speed travelling to Shop 3, 54 miles per hour, is faster than travelling to Shop 1. How long will it take her to drive to Shop 3?

ANSWER: A. 20 minutes

You know that Shop 3 is 20% farther away from Shop 1. As Shop 1 is located 15 miles away, Shop 3 is (15/100) × 120 = 18 miles away.

$$Time = \frac{Distance}{Speed} = \frac{18\ miles}{54\ miles\ per\ hour} = \frac{1}{3}\ hour = 20\ minutes$$

Although a seemingly awkward number, if you spotted that 54 is equal to 3 × 18 then you would quickly have seen that the answer is 1/3 of an hour, which is 20 minutes.

For the next questions, refer to **Example Set 3**. Allow yourself 160 seconds to complete the next four questions, making note of your answers before moving on to the explanations.

Example Set 3

Roger has gone to the supermarket to buy a ready-made lasagne. The price of Antonio's Amazing Lasagne is £5.35 per packet, while the Budget Lasagne is £4.00. He looks at the nutritional information of the two different packages:

Antonio's Amazing Lasagne		
	Per 100 g	**Per Quarter Pack**
Calories (kCal)	152	190
Fat (g)	7.4	9.25
– of which saturated fat (g)	3.6	4.5
Sugar (g)	4.0	5.0
Salt (g)	0.6	0.75
Budget Lasagne		
	Per 100 g	**Per Half Pack**
Calories (kCal)	200	600
Fat (g)	9.8	29.4
– of which saturated fat (g)	6.6	19.8
Sugar (g)	5.7	17.1
Salt (g)	0.8	2.4

1. What is the weight of one packet of Antonio's Amazing Lasagne?

    A.   125 g
    B.   400 g
    C.   500 g
    D.   600 g
    E.   Can't Tell

2. What percentage of the Budget Lasagne is made of fat?

    A.   6%
    B.   6.5%
    C.   10%
    D.   16.5%
    E.   Can't Tell

3. The Budget Lasagne weighs 600 g per pack. Roger has invited four friends for dinner and everyone, including him, will eat 300 g of lasagne. How much will it cost him if he buys them all Budget Lasagne?

    A.   £7.00
    B.   £8.00
    C.   £10.00
    D.   £12.00
    E.   £15.00

4. It transpires that there was a labelling error for the Budget Lasagne, and the calorie count was in fact 20% higher than labelled. How many calories are there per pack of Budget Lasagne?

    A.   720 kCal
    B.   1200 kCal
    C.   1320 kCal
    D.   1440 kCal
    E.   2880 kCal

Example Set 3: Answers and Explanations

Question 1

What is the weight of one packet of Antonio's Amazing Lasagne?

ANSWER: C. 500 g

On the surface, this question looks like it's not possible to answer. But you have been presented with values, both per 100 g and per quarter pack. You can therefore calculate the ratio between them. If you look at the sugar content of Antonio's Amazing Lasagne, you don't need a calculator to see that the 'per quarter' value is 125% of the 100 g value. Therefore, there are 1.25 multiples of 100 g in a quarter pack. So, a quarter pack must weigh 125 g. A full pack weighs 4 times a quarter pack, so 500 g.

Question 2

What percentage of the Budget Lasagne is made of fat?

ANSWER: C. 10%

This is an incredibly simple question to answer. Yet many struggle. You do not need to perform any calculations, as you have been presented with a percentage table in your data. You have all the values per 100 g. Anything per 100 is effectively synonymous with percentages. So all you have to do is read off the value which is 9.8%. Sometimes numbers are rounded slightly up or down. If this is the case you will almost certainly be presented with 'Can't Tell' as an answer option. But remember: 'Can't Tell' means it's *not possible* to calculate the answer; not that you disagree with the other options.

Question 3

The Budget Lasagne weighs 600 g per pack. Roger has invited four friends for dinner and everyone will eat 300 g of lasagne. How much will it cost him if he buys them all Budget Lasagne?

ANSWER: D. £12.00

As Roger is having four friends round for dinner, there will be five people eating in total: the four friends plus Roger himself. As each person eats 300 g of lasagne, he will need to buy 1500 g. The Budget Lasagne comes in packets of 600 g. So, he will need to buy three packets (1800 g), since he cannot buy half a packet. Therefore, the price is 3 × £4.00 = £12.00.

Question 4

It transpires that there was a labelling error for the Budget Lasagne, and the calorie count was in fact 20% higher than labelled. How many calories are there per pack of Budget Lasagne?

ANSWER: D. 1440 kCal

The original table told you that there were 600 kCal per half pack. With the labelling error, this means that there was in fact 720 kCal per half pack. For a full pack, you need to double this value, giving you 1440 kCal.

> **Top Tip:** When faced with recipe questions, remember that if you 'buy' something you must round up to the nearest whole integer, as you cannot buy fractions of items. However, if you 'use' an ingredient, you can work in fractions.

For the next questions, refer to **Example Set 4**. Allow yourself 160 seconds to complete the next four questions, making note of your answers before moving on to the explanations.

Example Set 4

Peter and Paul are both going on holiday and have decided to drive. Peter is driving from London to Frankfurt with an overnight stop in Paris. Paul is driving from London to Zurich, stopping in Paris for lunch. The distances between the cities (in miles) are:

	London	Paris	Frankfurt	Zurich
London	–	206	450	475
Paris	206	–	294	294
Frankfurt	450	294	–	183
Zurich	475	294	183	–

1. Peter leaves London at 17:35 arriving in Paris four hours later. The next morning he sets off at 09:15 and drives straight to Frankfurt, arriving at 15:15. What was his average speed?

    A. 45 miles per hour

    B. 50 miles per hour

    C. 52 miles per hour

    D. 56 miles per hour

    E. 60 miles per hour

2. While driving, Peter discovers the E50 connecting Paris to Frankfurt is shut due to an accident. He has to take a diversion, increasing his journey by 29.4 miles. By what percentage does his journey from Paris to Frankfurt increase?

    A. 4%

    B. 4.5%

    C. 5%

    D. 9%

    E. 10%

3. Paul drove at an average speed of 50 miles per hour. How long did it take him to get from London to Zurich?

   A.   9 hours

   B.   9.1 hours

   C.   9.5 hours

   D.   10 hours

   E.   Can't Tell

4. Peter's friend, Chris, is driving from Frankfurt to Zurich. His car has a petrol tank that can fit 60 litres of fuel and the price of petrol is £1.25 per litre. He uses 80% of a tank of petrol to make the journey. How much does the petrol for his journey cost?

   A.   £60.00

   B.   £75.00

   C.   £80.00

   D.   £90.00

   E.   £100.00

Example Set 4: Answers and Explanations

Question 1

Peter leaves London at 17:35 arriving in Paris four hours later. The next morning he sets off at 09:15 and drives straight to Frankfurt, arriving at 15:15. What was his average speed?

ANSWER: B. 50 miles per hour

This question again tests your knowledge of the equation: speed = distance/time. The distance is found using your table. London to Paris (206 miles) and Paris to Frankfurt (294 miles) gives a total of 500 miles. The time can easily be calculated: London to Paris (4 hours) and Paris to Frankfurt (6 hours) gives a total of 10 hours.

$$Speed = \frac{distance\,(500\;miles)}{time\,(10\;hours)} = 50\;miles\;per\;hour$$

Question 2

While driving, Peter discovers the E50 connecting Paris to Frankfurt is shut due to an accident. He has to take a diversion, increasing his journey by 29.4 miles. By what percentage does his journey from Paris to Frankfurt increase?

ANSWER: E. 10%

$$Percentage\;change = \frac{Difference}{Original}$$

Therefore, the percentage change = (29.4/294) × 100 = 10%

> **Top Tip:** When calculating percentage change it's easy, especially under time pressure, to divide the difference by the *final* value, instead of the *original* value. Always ensure you are using the original value, otherwise your answer will be wrong.

Question 3

Paul drove at an average speed of 50 miles per hour. How long did it take him to get from London to Zurich?

ANSWER: E. Can't Tell

It is tempting to rearrange the equation to give time = distance/speed. But this is incorrect. The introduction to the scenario tells you that Paul drove from London to Zurich, stopping in Paris for lunch. But you do not know how long he stopped in Paris. So how can you tell how long his journey took him?

> **Top Tip:** Always read the introductory text surrounding the data. It often contains crucial information required for the question!

Question 4

Peter's friend, Chris, is driving from Frankfurt to Zurich. His car has a petrol tank that can fit 60 litres of fuel and the price of petrol is £1.25 per litre. He uses 80% of a tank of petrol to make the journey. How much does the petrol for his journey cost?

ANSWER: A. £60

The cost of a full tank of fuel is £1.25 × 60 = £75.00. As Chris only requires 80% of a tank, the total cost is £75/100 × 80 = £60.00.

For the next questions, refer to **Example Set 5**. Allow yourself 160 seconds to complete the next four questions, making note of your answers before moving on to the explanations.

Example Set 5

A news agent is analysing his business and looks at the percentage of different items sold on different days during one week to improve his marketing campaign. The percentage of different items sold each day was plotted as follows:

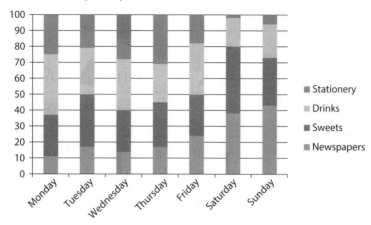

Perishable items are defined as those that may spoil, including drinks and sweets.

1. Which of the following pie charts represents the distribution of items sold on a Sunday?

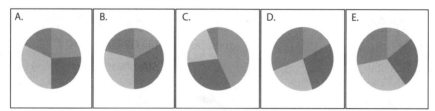

2. On the Wednesday he sold 280 items. How many sweets did he sell?

   A. 42

   B. 48

   C. 56

   D. 70

   E. 112

3. During the same week last year the newsagent sold 2480 items; however this year he sold 15% fewer items. How many items did he sell this week?

   A. 1984

   B. 2108

   C. 2356

   D. 2852

   E. 2976

4. On which day did he sell the most sweets?

   A.   Wednesday

   B.   Thursday

   C.   Friday

   D.   Saturday

   E.   Can't Tell

Example Set 5: Answers and Explanations

Question 1

Which of the following pie charts represents the distribution of items sold on a Sunday?

ANSWER: C

Looking at the data, you need to select the pie chart with the lowest proportion of stationery sold, as well as the highest proportion of newspapers. The only pie chart fitting this description is C.

Question 2

On the Wednesday he sold 280 items. How many sweets did he sell?

ANSWER: D. 70

In percentage-stacked charts the percentage contribution of an item is represented by the difference between the upper and lower values. As such, on Wednesday, sweet sales made up 40% – 15% (which was made up from newspaper sales) = 25%.

As the shop made a total of 280 sales, the number of sweets sold = (280/100) × 25 = 70.

Question 3

During the same week last year the newsagent sold 2480 items. However this year he sold 15% fewer items. How many items did he sell this week?

ANSWER: B. 2108

This is another example of a question testing the common percentage formula. As he sold 15% fewer items this year you know that he sold 85% of the total last year. So in other words, the question is asking what is 85% of 2480.

$$\frac{2480}{100} \times 85 = 2108 \text{ items}$$

Question 4

On which day did he sell the most sweets?

ANSWER: E. Can't Tell

This is a trick question. You have a stacked percentage chart, which shows the *percentage* of each item sold relative to the total. You do not, however, know how many items he sold each day. So, although proportionally he sold more sweets on the Saturday, you do not know what absolute value this correlates to. Therefore, the answer is 'Can't Tell'.

For the next questions, refer to **Example Set 6**. Allow yourself 160 seconds to complete the next four questions, making note of your answers before moving on to the explanations.

Example Set 6

Below is a symmetrical shape (not to scale). All measurements are in cm.

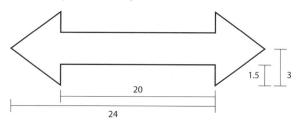

1. What is the area of the shape?

   A.   54 cm²

   B.   60 cm²

   C.   72 cm²

   D.   84 cm²

   E.   108 cm²

2. What is the perimeter of the shape?

   A.   46 cm

   B.   52 cm

   C.   54 cm

   D.   60 cm

   E.   66 cm

3. A symmetrical box has a volume of 64 cm³. What is the surface area of the box?

   A.   48 cm²

   B.   96 cm²

   C.   128 cm²

   D.   256 cm²

   E.   Can't Tell

4. A tropical fish enthusiast adds a new fish with a volume of 80 cm³ to his existing rectangular fish tank (20 × 20 × 10 cm), partly filled with 2000 cm³ of water. What is the percentage increase in the volume of the contents?

    A.   0.3%

    B.   0.7%

    C.   2.5%

    D.   3.5%

    E.   4%

Example Set 6: Answers and Explanations

Question 1

What is the area of the shape?

ANSWER: D. 84 cm²

Two-dimensional shapes are more common in UKCAT than three-dimensional shapes. Two-dimensional shapes tend to be semi-abstract, i.e. common shapes merged together.
To calculate the area of semi-abstract shapes, you need to divide them into their component parts. In this case, that's a rectangle and two triangles. To make life harder, the required measurements are often not present. When that happens, you will need to calculate them:

- The area of the rectangle is the width × length = 20 × 3 = 60 cm²
- The area of a right-angled triangle is ½ × base × height = ½ × 3 × 4 = 6
- As you have four right-angled triangles, their total area is 24 cm²
- Therefore, the total area is 84 cm²

Question 2

What is the perimeter of the shape?

ANSWER: E. 66 cm

If you divide the semi-abstract shape into its component parts, you will notice it is a rectangle with a triangle at either end. Each triangle can be subdivided into two right-angled triangles. You should hopefully see, without the need for Pythagoras' theorem, that the four right-angled triangles are '3, 4, 5 triangles'. As such, the hypotenuse is 5 cm.

When you add each side together (5 + 5 + 5 + 5 + 20 + 20 + 1.5 + 1.5 + 1.5 + 1.5) they total 66 cm.

Question 3

A symmetrical box has a volume of 64 cm³. What is the surface area of the box?

ANSWER: 96 cm²

As the box is symmetrical you know all sides are of equal length. The volume of a box is the length × height × width. Therefore, as each of these measurements has to be equal, each of the sides of the box is 4 cm in length (the cubed root of 64). The area of one side is therefore 16 cm² (width × length). As a box has six sides, the total surface area is 16 × 6 = 96 cm².

Question 4

A tropical fish enthusiast adds a new fish, with a volume of 80 cm³, to his existing rectangular fish tank (20 × 20 × 10 cm), partly filled with 2000 cm³ of water. What is the percentage increase in the volume of the contents?

ANSWER: E. 4%

More information is provided than is required. Remember the percentage change formula from earlier: Percentage change = difference/original value × 100. So in this case: 80/2000 × 100 = 4%.

Summary of Quantitative Reasoning

Remember: The Quantitative Reasoning section of the UKCAT is less to do with maths, and more to do with logical reasoning. This cannot be emphasised enough! It is possible to do the vast majority, if not all, of the QR questions without the use of a calculator. The on-screen calculator is cumbersome and awkward to use, not to mention time consuming. So avoid it if you can!

There are a few formulae that come up frequently, and which you should know well:

$$Speed = \frac{Distance}{Time}$$

$$Percentage = \left(\frac{Given\ amount}{Total\ amount}\right) \times 100$$

$$Percentage\ change = \left(\frac{Difference}{Original}\right) \times 100$$

$$Average = \frac{Sum\ of\ numbers}{Number\ of\ numbers}$$

Mode: The most commonly occurring value

Median: The middle value in a data set

In addition to the above, there are some basic geometrical formulas to be aware of:

Two-Dimensional Shapes		
Shape	Perimeter	Area
Square	4 S	S^2
Rectangle	$(2 \times L) + (2 \times H)$	$L \times H$
Parallelogram	S1 + S2 + S3 + S4	$B \times H$
Circle	$2\pi r$ or πd	πr^2
Triangle	A + B + C	$\frac{1}{2} \times B \times H$

Three-Dimensional Shapes		
Shape	Surface Area	Volume
Box	2lw + 2lh + 2wh	$l \times w \times h$
Sphere	$4\pi r^2$	$4/3\ \pi r^3$
Cylinder	$2\pi r(r + h)$	$\pi r^2 h$

N.B.: Although knowledge to 'the standard of a good pass at GCSE' requires you to know that $\pi = 3.14$, it is very rare that QR questions require you to work with π as an absolute number. You do get questions relating to circles and, more rarely, spheres and cylinders. But in these cases, the questions tend to be designed in such a way that they express π as part of the answer, not as an absolute number.

Time for some practice! Try answering the following nine **Practice Sets**. You have 24 minutes to answer all questions. Detailed explanations are provided. Good luck!

Practice Sets

Scenario 1

Two friends, Matthew and John, have decided to race each other on bikes around the woods. They have set up three checkpoints: A, B and C. They both start at point A, with Matthew cycling from A to B to C then back to A. John, however, is cycling from A to C to B to A. The distance from A to B is 4 miles and from B to C is 6 miles. It takes Matthew 20 minutes to cycle from A to B and he completes the entire course in 90 minutes. Matthew arrives back at point A half an hour before John.

Question 1: How much faster did Matthew cycle compared with John?

    A. 25%

    B. One-third

    C. 4/9

    D. 0.75

    E. Can't tell

Question 2: Assuming Matthew cycles at a constant speed throughout, how far is it between points C and A?

    A. 4 miles

    B. 6 miles

    C. 8 miles

    D. 10 miles

    E. 18 miles

Question 3: After the race it transpired that John had gotten lost between points C and B, increasing his race distance. In total John cycled 22 miles. What was his average speed?

    A. 11 miles per hour

    B. 12 miles per hour

    C. 13 miles per hour

    D. 14 miles per hour

    E. 15 miles per hour

Question 4: The friends decide that, as cycling is very good for keeping fit, burning approximately 500 kCal per hour, they should do two hours a week cycling for all but four weeks in the year. How many calories per year will they each burn as a result?

    A. 24,000 Cal

    B. 26,000 Cal

    C. 48,000 Cal

    D. 52,000 Cal

    E. 48,000,000 Cal

Scenario 2

James is currently driving to and from his office every Monday to Friday but feels it's time to upgrade to a new car. He is undecided about which car to get so he has created the table below:

	Audi A4	Audi A5	Mercedes C Class
Price	£23,600	£28,670	£24,450
Engine size	2.0 L	1.8 L	1.8 L
0 – 60 mph	9.2 s	7.6 s	8.7 s
Horsepower	134 BHP	167 BHP	153 BHP
Top speed	134 mph	143 mph	140 mph

Question 1: If James wishes to upgrade the sound system on the Audi A5 he needs to pay an additional £716.75. What is the percentage increase in total price?

    A. 2%

    B. 2.25%

    C. 2.5%

    D. 2.75%

    E. 3%

Question 2: To buy the Audi A4, James takes out a loan. The terms of the loan require him to pay a 25% deposit followed by 24 monthly payments of £800. How much extra will James have to pay above list price?

    A. £1400

    B. £1475

    C. £1500

    D. £1625

    E. £2767.50

Question 3: The Mercedes C Class has a fuel tank size of 67.5 litres and a fuel economy of 40 miles per gallon. One gallon is approximately 4.5 litres. How far can the Mercedes C Class travel on 1/3 of a tank of petrol?

    A. 182.25 miles

    B. 200 miles

    C. 300 miles

    D. 400 miles

    E. 600 miles

Question 4: James commutes 25 miles to work every day. If he bought the Audi A4, his fuel efficiency would be 10 miles per litre of petrol. Currently, petrol costs £1.40 per litre. How much would it cost him to commute to and from work every week?

    A. £17.50

    B. £26.25

    C. £35.00

    D. £49.00

    E. Can't Tell

Scenario 3

Noradrenaline is a drug used in critical care units to increase the blood pressure of patients in shock. It has to be given as a continuous infusion, the strength of which varies as standard strength (4 mg of noradrenaline diluted in 50 mL of saline), double strength (8 mg of noradrenaline diluted in 50 mL saline) and quadruple strength (16 mg noradrenaline diluted in 50 mL saline).

Question 1: A patient is receiving an infusion of standard strength noradrenaline at a rate of 0.5 micrograms per kilogram of body weight per minute. He weighs 70 kg. How much noradrenaline is he receiving per hour?

    A. 21 mcg

    B. 35 mcg

    C. 2.1 mg

    D. 35 mg

    E. 2.1 g

Question 2: A 60-year-old man weighing 62.5 kg is requiring 3 mg noradrenaline per hour. How many syringes of double-strength noradrenaline will he require per 24 hours?

    A. 3

    B. 5

    C. 6

    D. 9

    E. 18

Question 3: Noradrenaline is sold in vials containing 4 mg of powder each, costing £11.55 per vial. Saline costs £0.10 per 10 mL container. To draw up the solution, staff require a 50-mL syringe (costing £0.45) and a needle (costing £0.12). What is the cost of drawing up a quadruple strength noradrenaline infusion?

    A. £12.22

    B. £12.62

    C. £24.17

D. £46.87

E. £47.27

Question 4: The average cost per night for a patient staying in an intensive care unit is £1500. The intensive care unit at a district general hospital has eight beds, and runs at an average occupancy of 75% throughout the year. What is the annual cost of patients staying in the intensive care unit?

A. £2,190,000

B. £3,285,000

C. £3,832,500

D. £4,380,000

E. Can't Tell

Scenario 4

It's Jane's 12th birthday party and her parents are planning on ordering pizza. They've invited 24 of Jane's friends, along with two other parents to help out. On average, each adult will eat five slices of pizza, while each child will eat three slices. To keep it simple, they will order an equal number of meat and vegetarian pizzas.

Question 1: Assuming each pizza has eight slices, how many pizzas do they need to order?

A. 10

B. 11

C. 12

D. 13

E. Can't Tell

Question 2: The cost of a vegetarian pizza is £12; however, the meat pizza is 1/3 more expensive. What is the cost per slice of the meat pizza?

A. £0.50

B. £1.00

C. £2.00

D. £8.00

E. £16.00

Question 3: The radius of a large (eight-slice) pizza is 15 cm, while the radius of a small pizza is 5 cm. How many times larger is the area of the large pizza as compared to the small pizza?

A. 3

B. 9

C. 10

D. 12

E. Can't Tell

Question 4: Last year when they ordered pizza for Jane's 11th birthday her parents spent £150.00 including delivery. This year, however, the total bill came to £157.50. What is the percentage increase in cost of the food bill?

    A. 5%

    B. 7.5%

    C. 10%

    D. 15%

    E. Can't Tell

Scenario 5

White blood cells are produced by the body to fight infection. There are five main types of white blood cell that collectively make up the total white blood cell count. These five cell types are neutrophils, leucocytes, monocytes, eosinophils and basophils. Following is a table of blood results of three patients:

	Normal Values	Patient 1	Patient 2	Patient 3
Haemoglobin (g/dL)	13 to 17	10.4	13.8	14.3
White Cell Count ($\times 10^9$/L) Total Neutrophils Leucocytes	3 to 10 2 to 7.5 1.5 to 4	15.8 8.9 5.3	22.5 15.3 2.7	13.3 11.2 1.5
Platelets ($\times 10^9$/L)	150 to 400	155	440	330

Question 1: What proportion of the white blood cells is made up of cells other than neutrophils and leucocytes in patient 2?

    A. 1/3

    B. 1/4

    C. 1/5

    D. 1/6

    E. Can't Tell

Question 2: When they repeated the blood tests the next day, the platelet count of patient 3 had decreased by 20%. What was his platelet count the next day?

    A. 124

    B. 264

    C. 297

    D. 332

    E. 396

Question 3: The estimated blood volume of patient 1 is 6 L. How many grams of haemoglobin does his blood contain?

    A. 624

    B. 1040

    C. 3120

    D. 6240

    E. 8280

Question 4: Patient 2 is treated with the antibiotic meropenam, costing £10 per half gram. He requires 0.5 g of meropenam three times per day for 7 days. This 7-day course costs six times as much as a standard 5-day course of the antibiotic erythromycin. How much does a standard 5-day course of erythromycin cost per day?

    A. £5.00

    B. £7.00

    C. £14.00

    D. £35.00

    E. £70.00

Scenario 6

Mike and Sarah are buying a house together. On the ground floor there are two reception rooms (3 m x 6 m) and (4 m x 7 m), a kitchen/diner (5 m x 4 m) and a hallway. The hallway is 1/4 of the size of the largest reception room.

Question 1: What is the surface area of the ground floor?

    A. 66 m²

    B. 73 m²

    C. 77 m²

    D. 79 m²

    E. Can't Tell

Question 2: After buying the house they build a semicircular conservatory extension to the kitchen/diner, increasing the overall area of the kitchen/diner by 50%. To the nearest half metre, what is the diameter of the conservatory?

    A. 2.5 m

    B. 3 m

    C. 5 m

    D. 6 m

    E. Can't Tell

Question 3: Mike and Sarah bought their first house in 2013 for £225,000. It has subsequently increased in value by 6%. What is the value of their house today?

    A. £234,000

    B. £236,250

C. £238,500

D. £240,750

E. £265,000

Question 4: Mike and Sarah's friends, Archie and Abbey, are looking to buy their first house and are offered a mortgage allowing them to borrow 4 times their deposit. Archie has been saving 15% of his £60,000 per year salary as a chartered accountant for the last 5 years. They have put down a deposit on a £340,000 house. Abbey has only been saving for 2 years but contributed 25% of her salary annually. How much does Abbey earn per year?

A. £46,000

B. £80,000

C. £85,000

D. £92,000

E. £160,000

Scenario 7

Nina and Paul want to go from London to Tahiti for their honeymoon. They will be staying in a villa costing £500 per night. There are no direct flights for the 9500-mile journey via Los Angeles. After doing some online research, Paul has narrowed it down to two flight options:

Option 1:

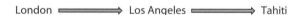

London ⟹ Los Angeles ⟹ Tahiti

Price per person: Economy £1495; Business Class £5600

Stopover in Los Angeles: 3 hours 55 minutes

Total journey time: 23 hours 55 minutes

Option 2:

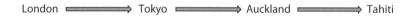

London ⟹ Tokyo ⟹ Auckland ⟹ Tahiti

Price per person: Economy £1355; Business Class £4750

Stop over in Tokyo: 1 hour 10 minutes

Stopover in Auckland: 2 hours 55 minutes

Total journey time: 33 hours 20 minutes

If they take option 1 they will arrive late on a Monday evening, whereas if they take option 2, they arrive early on the Tuesday morning and will only be able to stay for 9 nights in total.

Question 1: If they travel in business class via Tokyo, what is the cost of Nina and Paul's honeymoon?

A. £9250

B. £9750

C. £14,000

D. £14,500

E. £19,400

Question 2: If they travel using option 1, what is the average speed of the aircrafts?

A. 405 miles per hour

B. 475 miles per hour

C. 488 miles per hour

D. 500 miles per hour

E. Can't Tell

Question 3: The time zone in Tahiti (THAT) is 10 hours behind the UK (GMT). If Nina and Paul leave at 13:45 GMT on a Wednesday from London using flight option 2, when, in local time, do they arrive in Tahiti?

A. 12:45 on Thursday

B. 13:05 on Thursday

C. 23:05 on Thursday

D. 13:05 on Friday

E. 23:05 on Friday

Question 4: Before leaving, Nina and Paul decide to exchange 500 pounds (GBP) into US dollars (USD) at an exchange rate of 1 GBP = 1.60 USD. When exchanging the currency, the agency takes 4% in commission. How much do they pay in commission?

A. 20 USD

B. 32 USD

C. 40 USD

D. 768 USD

E. 780 USD

Scenario 8

John has bought an empty glass aquarium with an open top and plans on keeping exotic fish. Below is a diagram of the aquarium he bought, which measures 20 × 10 × 10 cm:

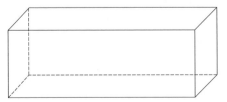

Question 1: John fills the aquarium 3/4 of the way to the top with 2 parts hot to 1 part cold water to reach the desired temperature. What volume of cold water does he add?

A. 500 cm³

B. 750 cm³

C. 1000 cm³

D. 1500 cm³

E. 2000 cm³

Question 2: What is the total surface area of the aquarium?

A. 800 cm²

B. 1000 cm²

C. 1600 cm²

D. 2000 cm²

E. Can't Tell

Question 3: When visiting the fish shop, large fish cost £12.50 each and small fish are priced at four for £5. How many times more expensive is a large fish compared with a small fish?

A. 2.5

B. 3

C. 5

D. 6

E. 10

Question 4: On a hot day the water temperature increases by 2°C to 27°C. What is the percentage increase in the water temperature?

A. 7.4%

B. 8%

C. 13.5%

D. 15%

E. Can't Tell

Scenario 9

While studying for his PhD in public health a student looked at mortality rates in two different countries: Country 1 and Country 2. He documented the cause of death for the first 30,000 patients who died that year, plotting the absolute number of deaths per condition. When plotting the data, respiratory disease was subdivided into acute (pneumonia) and chronic (COPD).

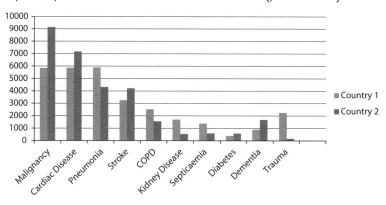

Question 1: How many people died of respiratory disease in Country 1?

    A. 2,525

    B. 5,884

    C. 5,895

    D. 8,391

    E. 14,235

Question 2: For which disease is the second biggest relative difference between the two countries?

    A. Kidney disease

    B. Pneumonia

    C. Septicaemia

    D. Dementia

    E. Trauma

Question 3: The student also looked at Country 3, which has a population of 10 million and a death rate of 800 per 100,000 people per year last year. The largest cause of death in Country 3 is cardiac disease, accounting for 1 in 4 deaths. How many people died of cardiac disease last year?

    A. 2,000

    B. 20,000

    C. 8,000

    D. 80,000

    E. Can't Tell

Question 4: A new screening technique for bowel cancer will be adopted in Country 2 next year, predicted to reduce malignancy related deaths by one-third. How many people will be predicted to die of a malignancy-related cause in Country 2 next year, assuming the other causes remain proportionally the same?

    A. 1948

    B. 3049

    C. 3896

    D. 6098

    E. Can't Tell

Answers

Scenario 1

Question 1: B. One-third

This is a simple question, but tests your knowledge of fractions and decimals and your ability to quickly convert between them.

Matthew finishes the race in 90 minutes while John takes 120 minutes (you are told he finishes 30 minutes after Matthew): 120/90 = 1.333*

Therefore Matthew cycles one-third faster than John.

Question 2: C. 8 miles

This is a three-step calculation. You need to calculate:

1. Matthew's average speed: distance/time = 4 miles/20 minutes = 12 mph.
2. Total distance travelled: you are told he cycles at a constant speed and the total time spent is 90 minutes. Therefore, travelling at 12 mph he covers a total distance of 18 miles.
3. Subtract A to B and B to C from the total distance = 18 – 6 – 4 = 8 miles.

Question 3: A. 11 miles per hour

Remember the formula:

$$Speed = \frac{Distance}{Time} = \frac{22}{2} = 11\,mph$$

Question 4: E. 48,000,000 Cal

There are 52 weeks in a year and they plan to cycle all but 4. Therefore, they will cycle 48 times per year. On each occasion they plan to cycle for 2 hours, which gives a total of 96 hours per year. At 500 kCal per hour, this gives 48,000 kCal per year.

Remember your units:

Kilo × 1,000

Mega × 1,000,000

The answers are in Cal, not kCal; therefore you have to convert 48,000 kCal to Cal by multiplying by 1000.

Scenario 2

Question 1: C. 2.5%

$$Percentage\ change = \frac{difference}{original\ number} \times 100$$
$$= \frac{716.75}{28670} \times 100 = 2.5\%$$

Question 2: C. £1500

Step 1: Calculate the total James will have to pay = deposit + monthly payments

$$\left(\frac{23600}{4}\right)+(24\times800)=5900+19200=25100$$

Step 2: Subtract the price from the paid price.

$$=25100-23600=£1500$$

Remember, the question asks about the price of the Audi A4, *not* the A5 as in the previous question.

Question 3: B. 200 miles

Step 1: Calculate the size of the petrol tank in gallons.

$$=\frac{67.5}{4.5}=15$$

Step 2: Calculate how far you can drive on a third of a tank of petrol.

$$=\frac{(40\times15)}{3}=\frac{600}{3}=200\ miles$$

Question 4: C. £35.00

Step 1: Calculate the total commute.

The total commute is the distance per day (25 miles x 2) multiplied by the number of days per week driven (5, as it states clearly in the opening section of the question) = 250 miles

Step 2: Calculate the number of litres of petrol required.

$$=\frac{250}{10}=25$$

Step 3: Calculate the total cost of petrol.

$$=25\times1.40=£35.00$$

Scenario 3

Question 1: C. 2.1 mg

The amount of noradrenaline received per minute is 0.5 x 70 = 35 mcg. Multiply this by 60 to get the amount per hour = 2100 mcg. This is not an available answer but remember your units! 1 milligram = 1000 microgram; therefore 2100 microgram = 2.1 milligram. Equally, looking at the answers, you could quickly eliminate A and B as they are the wrong order of magnitude, as is E.

Question 2: D. 9

This is a two-step calculation. First you need to calculate how much noradrenaline he requires per 24 hours (step 1), then work out how many syringes of *double*-strength noradrenaline this is.

Step 1: 24 x 3 mg = 72 mg

Step 2: 72/8 = 9 (remember there are 8 mg per syringe of double-strength noradrenaline)

Question 3: E. £47.27

This is a straightforward question provided you use the right numbers! To make the solution you will require 16 mg of noradrenaline (4 vials at £11.55 each), 50 mL of saline (5 × 10 mL saline containers at £0.10 each), a syringe (£0.45) and a needle (£0.12).

Total price = (11.55 × 4) + (0.1 × 5) + 0.45 + 0.12 = £47.27

Question 4: B. £3,285,000

Step 1: Calculate the number of 'bed nights per year':

$$= 75\% \text{ of } (365 \times 8) = \left(\frac{2920}{100}\right) \times 75 = 2190 \text{ nights}$$

Step 2: Calculate the total cost:

$$= 2190 \times 1500 = £3,285,000$$

Scenario 4

Question 1: C. 12

There will be a total of 25 children (Jane and 24 friends) and 4 adults (Jane's parents and 2 other parents). As each child eats 3 slices and each adult 5 slices they will need a total of 75 + 20 = 95 slices. This equates to 11.875 pizzas. As you can't order 0.875 pizzas they will need to order 12 pizzas.

Question 2: C. £2.00

12 + (12/3) = £16 per pizza. As each pizza has 8 slices, this equates to £2.00 per slice.

Question 3: B. 9

The area of a circle is πr^2. The large pizza is 3 times larger than the small pizza. When rearranging the formula, 3^2 is 9, therefore the area of the large pizza is 9 times that of the small pizza.

Question 4: A. 5%

Percentage change is (Difference/Original) × 100. Therefore: (7.50/150) × 100 = 5.

Scenario 5

Question 1: C. 1/5

Step 1: Work out how many blood cells make up the remaining cells other than neutrophils and leucocytes:

Total – (neutrophils + leucocytes) = 22.5 – (15.3 + 2.7) = 4.5

Step 2: Calculate the ratio:

22.5:4.5 = 5:1

Question 2: B. 264

All you need to do is calculate 80% of the original platelet count of patient 3:

$$\frac{330}{100} \times 80 = 264$$

Alternatively, you can quickly calculate that 10% is 33; therefore 20% is 66.

$$330 - 66 = 264$$

Question 3: A. 624 g

Step 1: The table tells you that the value of haemoglobin is in grams per decilitre. Remember, there are 10 decilitres in 1 litre; therefore, there are 60 decilitres in 6 L (the blood volume of patient 1).

Step 2: Calculate the weight of haemoglobin.

$$60 \times 10.4 = 624 \text{ g}$$

Question 4: B. £7.00

Step 1: Calculate the cost of a 7-day course of meropenam:

$$\left(\frac{£20}{2}\right) \times 3 \times 7 = £210$$

Step 2: Calculate the total cost of a 5-day course of erythromycin:

$$\frac{210}{6} = £35$$

Step 3: Calculate the cost per day of erythromycin:

$$\frac{35}{5} = £7$$

Scenario 6

Question 1: B. 73 m²

The total surface area is: $(6 \times 3) + (4 \times 7) + (4 \times 5) + (28/4) = 73 \text{ m}^2$.

Question 2: C. 5 m

The current kitchen/diner is 20 m², so the area of the conservatory is 10 m².

The area of a semi-circle is $(\pi r^2)/2$. Therefore $(\pi r^2)/2 = 10$. This gives $\pi r^2 = 20$.

$$r^2 = \frac{20}{\pi} = 6.37$$

Therefore $r = \sqrt{6.37} = 2.5 \text{ m}$.

Remember the diameter is twice the radius! Therefore the diameter is 5 m.

Question 3: C. £238,500

This is a simple calculation:

$$\left(\frac{225,000}{100}\right) \times 106 = £238,500$$

Question 4: A. £46,000

There are several calculations to perform quickly.

Step 1: Calculate the deposit contributed by Archie:

$$\left[\left(\frac{60,000}{100}\right)\times 15\right]\times 5 = £45,000$$

Step 2: Calculate the total deposit placed:

$$\frac{340,000}{5} = £68,000$$

Step 3: Calculate Abbey's share:

$$68,000 - 45,000 = £23,000$$

Step 4: Abbey's salary = 23,000/2 = £11,500 per year of contributions, which is 25% of her salary. Therefore her salary = £11,500 ×4 = £46,000 per year.

Scenario 7

Question 1: C. £14,000

The total price is the flight + hotel stay.

$flight = £4,750 \times 2$ (as two people travelling)

$accommodation = £500 \times 9$ (last sentence says if taking option 2 can only stay 9 nights)

Total price is 9500 + 4500 = £14,000.

Question 2: B. 475 miles per hour

Use the formula speed = distance/time.

Distance is 9500 miles and the time in the air is calculated as the total travel time with the stop-over times subtracted:

23 hours 55 minutes $- 3$ hours 55 minutes $= 20$ hours

$$Speed = \frac{9500}{20} = 475 \text{ miles per hour}$$

Question 3: B. 13:05 Thursday

The total journey time for option 2 is 33 hours and 20 minutes. If they leave London at 13:45 on Wednesday, they will arrive at 23:05 GMT Thursday. As Tahiti is 10 hours behind the UK, this is 13:05 Thursday.

Question 4: B. 32 USD

The first step is to calculate how many USD they will receive:

$USD = 500 \times 1.6 = 800 \text{ USD}$

Then you can calculate the commission (which is 4%):

$$\frac{800}{100} \times 4 = 32 \text{ USD}$$

Scenario 8

Question 1: A. 500 cm³

The volume of a box can be calculated as:

$l \times w \times h = 20 \times 10 \times 10 = 2000 \ cm^3$

As he fills the aquarium 3/4 to the top with water, he adds 1500 cm³ water. This is added in a ratio of 2:1 hot to cool. He therefore adds 1/3 of the water as cold water = 500 cm³.

Question 2: A. 800 cm²

The trick in this question is that the introduction told you the aquarium has an open top. Therefore, you cannot add this area to the total. It is therefore:

$3 \times (20 \times 10) + 2(10 \times 10) = 800 \ cm^2$

Question 3: E. 10

The price of one small fish is £1.25 (as you buy 4 for £5). As the large fish costs £12.50 this is 10 times the price of a small fish.

Question 4: B. 8%

You know that the water temperature increases by 2°C; therefore, the original temperature must have been 25°C.

$$percentage \ change = \frac{difference}{original} \times 100 = \frac{2}{25} \times 100 = 8$$

Scenario 9

Question 1: D. 8391

The introductory paragraph stated that the definition of respiratory disease was acute (pneumonia) and chronic (COPD) combined. As such, you will need to total the relevant value from each column for Country 1.

It is impossible to see the exact numbers, but looking at the tables the values are roughly 5900 for pneumonia and 2500 for COPD = 8400.

As 'Can't Tell' is not an option, you need to look at the closest matching answer; in this case D (8391). As none of the others are close, they are not possible.

Question 2: A. Kidney disease

For this question you need to look at the proportions between the columns for the two countries for each disease and find the one with the *second* biggest difference. Clearly the biggest difference between the countries is for trauma (approximately 13 times), while the second biggest difference is for kidney disease (approximately 3 times more in Country 1 compared with Country 2).

The answer can be found by looking at your data. Septicaemia, however, does look very similar, but the absolute values are lower in Country 1 and higher in Country 2 compared with the absolute values for kidney disease. The relative proportion must therefore be lower (in this case approximately double only).

Question 3: B. 20,000

This is a two-step calculation.

Step 1: Find the absolute numbers of deaths last year:

$$800 \times \left(\frac{10,000,000}{100,000} \right) = 80,000$$

Step 2: Calculate the number of cardiac-related deaths:

$$\frac{80,000}{4} = 20,000$$

Question 4: E. Can't Tell

Looking at the table, Country 2 has just over 9000 malignancy-associated deaths in the first 35,000 deaths last year. So this would represent a reduction of approximately 3000 deaths in this group, resulting in approximately 6000 malignancy related deaths in total.

However, the data given states it is for the first 35,000 deaths per year. You do not know how many total deaths there actually are per year in Country 2, nor the population size or mortality rates, so you cannot calculate the absolute number for the whole country.

CHAPTER 3

Abstract Reasoning

Overview

Abstract Reasoning (AR) tests your ability to recognise patterns among distracting material. It does this by asking you to say whether 'test shapes' fit into certain patterns. The UKCAT has also recently introduced a new style of AR question. This requires you to identify sequences and changes in patterns before choosing which shape should come next.

Format of the Section

You will be presented with 55 questions. These need to be answered in just 14 minutes (of which 1 minute is reading time). Although this works out as just over 14 seconds per question, many questions will be presented in sets of five. In this case, it's best to think of it as 70 seconds per question set.

There are four question types in AR:

- **Type 1:** You are presented with two 'sets' of shapes (Set A and Set B) followed by five 'test shapes'. You need to decide if the test shape fits into Set A, Set B or neither set.

- **Type 2:** This is a logical test, where you are presented with a series of shapes, alternating from one box to the next. You need to say which of four shapes would come next.

- **Type 3:** This is similar to Type 2, but instead of a series you are presented with a 'statement' where changes have been applied to one shape to create a new one. You must then apply the same changes to your test shape, and choose which of four options comes next.

- **Type 4:** A variation on Type 1 questions, but instead of five sequential 'test shapes' you are presented with four 'test shapes' simultaneously and have to decide which one of the four belongs to either Set A or B.

Students often find Type 2 and Type 3 questions easier than Type 1 or Type 4. This is mainly because these question types require *logical* thinking, rather than pure *spatial* reasoning – a skill that scientifically and mathematically minded students prefer.

Type 1 Questions

In Type 1 questions you will be presented with two sets of shapes: Set A and Set B. Each set is made up of six square boxes, and each of these boxes contains a pattern. The pattern will be consistent throughout the six boxes in the same set, but will be different in Set A and Set B. You will then be presented with five test shapes, one after the other, and asked if the test shape fits into Set A, Set B or neither set.

Demonstration Set

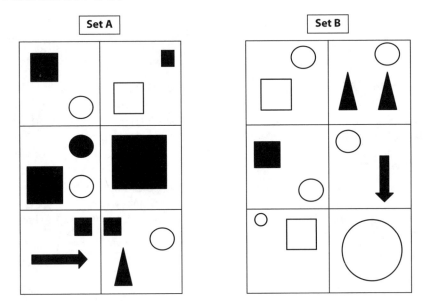

To which of the following sets do the test shapes below belong?

Test Shapes:

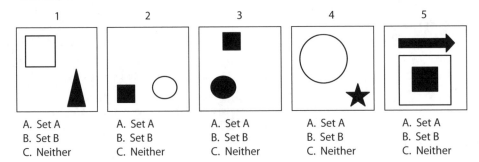

1	2	3	4	5
A. Set A	A. Set A	A. Set A	A. Set A	A. Set A
B. Set B	B. Set B	B. Set B	B. Set B	B. Set B
C. Neither	C. Neither	C. Neither	C. Neither	C. Neither

Answer Definitions

Set A

The test shape must match the pattern in all the boxes in Set A.

Set B

The test shape must match the pattern in all the boxes in Set B.

Neither

The test shape does *not* completely fit into either Set A or B.

OR

The test shape fits into *both* Set A and Set B (so there is no way to discriminate between the two answers).

Strategy

In order to identify the pattern and successfully answer the questions in the tight time constraint it is essential that you stick to a strategy, adopting an efficient technique to identify the patterns.

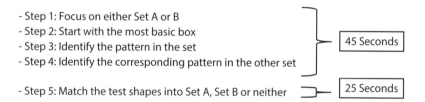

- Step 1: Focus on either Set A or B
- Step 2: Start with the most basic box
- Step 3: Identify the pattern in the set
- Step 4: Identify the corresponding pattern in the other set

45 Seconds

- Step 5: Match the test shapes into Set A, Set B or neither

25 Seconds

Step 1

It doesn't matter which set you start with. Ultimately, you will need to identify the patterns in both Set A and Set B in order to match your test shapes. If you are struggling to identify the pattern in Set A then focus on Set B. The patterns will be linked. Once you know what you're looking for (having identified the pattern in either Set A or B), you can apply those same rules to the opposite set. Hopefully, it should be easy to identify the second pattern.

Step 2

Identifying the pattern can be challenging. So here's a basic first trick to help you along. When assessing either Set A or B, look for the box containing the least number of items. In other words: the most basic box. Remember, the pattern has to be present in all six boxes of a set. It is easier to identify the pattern if there are fewer items to process.

Start by finding the most basic box in each set:

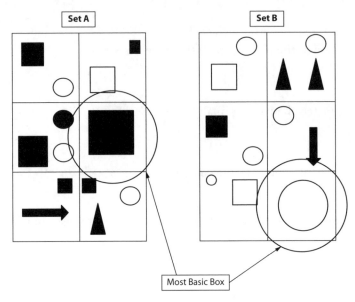

The above is a simplified example. It demonstrates that finding the pattern is much easier when there are fewer items to assess. However, this technique has two limiting factors:

1. What if there is no 'most basic' box?

2. You still might not be able to identify the pattern.

Steps 3 and 4

Identifying the pattern(s) is the most challenging part of the question. There seems to be infinite possible combinations. However, certain themes are more common than others. Patterns can be categorised in two ways:

- Non-conditional
- Conditional

Non-conditional patterns occur when the themes are independent, and do not depend on each other. Common examples include number of items, sides, angles, intersections etc. There may be several non-conditional patterns present in each set, but they are intrinsically linked between Set A and Set B. (Otherwise it would be impossible to identify all patterns in just 45 seconds.)

Conditional patterns occur when one of the themes is dependent on another. Students often find these tricky. For instance, the pattern might be: If the triangle points up in Set A, then there will be an odd number of small squares in the box; if it points down, then the number of small squares is even.

In Type 1 questions, you have just over 70 seconds per question set. You should therefore allow yourself up to 45 seconds to identify the patterns in Set A and B. This leaves you with 25 seconds to match your test shapes to the correct set.

It is imperative that you keep an eye on the timer! If you have not found the pattern within 45 seconds, you must select answers according to your gut instinct, 'flag' the question, and move on. Otherwise, you risk running out of time to complete the AR section. If you have time to spare after completing the section you can then attempt flagged questions again.

Step 5

Once you have identified the patterns in Set A and Set B, it is relatively quick to match your test shapes with the correct set. The process of assessing the test shape, matching it to the correct set and moving to the next question should take around 5 seconds.

Distractors

Abstract reasoning involves identifying patterns that are disguised among superfluous material. Within the boxes, there are often numerous items that do not contribute to the overall pattern. Rather, they *mask* the pattern by distracting you. These are the so-called 'distractors'. Until you know what the pattern is, you will not be able to identify which items are distractors and which contribute to the actual pattern. Distractors can therefore make it significantly harder to identify the underlying pattern.

Once you know what the pattern is, you can identify which items are distractors. In the following example, the simple pattern is a shaded square in every box of Set A. With this in mind, you can appreciate the distractors at work.

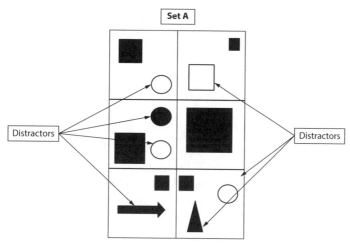

Troubleshooting

You might have trouble finding the pattern, in which case, try the following:

1. Move around! Some patterns are easier to see close up. Others are more obvious the farther away you are. 'Big picture' patterns, such as position and colour distribution, are easy to overlook when sitting close to the screen. So, if you're struggling, it is a good idea to move around and change your perspective.

2. Focus on both sets. The patterns between Set A and Set B are linked. Therefore, if you can't find the pattern in Set A, focus on Set B. Once you have identified a pattern in one set, you can apply the theme to the other. Hopefully, you will then find the pattern easily.

3. If you still can't find the pattern and you have used your 45 seconds then you must *move on*. It is easy to become engrossed in finding patterns. Before you know it, several minutes can pass. This makes it impossible to finish the rest of the section in time.

Patterns

There are a wide range of potential patterns but a few common patterns crop up regularly. Although it seems tough, students often report that Abstract Reasoning was the only section of the exam that was easier than expected!

Examples of common patterns include:

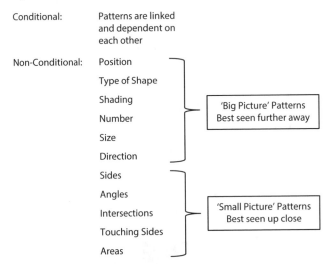

It is advisable to look for at least two patterns per set. Although there will be some difficult questions, which may feature more patterns, finding at least two patterns will allow you to get the correct answer in the majority of questions. After you have identified what the pattern relates to, e.g. right angles, you need to figure out how exactly it works. Considering the following two possibilities will help with this process:

*   Absolute numbers: What is the absolute number of a particular item/theme in each set?
*   Odd/even: Is there an odd number of a particular theme in one set, and an even number in the other?

Top Tip: If you spot a pattern falling into the odd/even category, always consider the possibility of a second pattern being present. Otherwise, the pattern would be too simple and 'Neither' will never be a viable answer option.

To help you hone in on key patterns, we have developed the **Impression Technique**. When you start a question and look at Set A and Set B you will get an 'impression' of the overall pattern. This impression is non-specific. It might be: 'Everything looks the same!' Or, simply: 'How random!'

Most questions give candidates one of seven 'impressions'. For each impression, there are a limited number of possible patterns to look for. If you can remember what patterns relate to each impression, this allows you to perform a much more systematic and focused search. This, in turn, improves your chances of successfully identifying the pattern.

The Impression Technique

When you first look at a question there are a number of different 'impressions' you might get. Broadly speaking, these fall into seven categories. For each impression there are a number of commonly occurring patterns to look for. Although there are exceptions, the majority of the time if you know what you're looking for then suddenly the 'hunt' becomes much easier. Memorizing what to look for in each impression will help you perform a structured search of the most commonly occurring patterns.

The seven categories that we have divided the impressions into are:

1. Everything looks the same

2. Different blocks of shapes

3. Arrows by themselves

4. Letters and words

5. Familiar objects

6. Abstract patterns

7. Something's changing

In addition to the above, there are also three **Special Circumstances** where rarely occurring events will offer clues to the correct pattern:

1. Items touching the side

2. Items overlapping

3. Arrows pointing to/from items

We will now work our way through numerous examples, looking at the different impressions and the potential patterns with which they are associated.

Refer to **Example Set 1** below. Set a timer for 70 seconds and make a note of your answers before moving on to the explanations.

Example Set 1

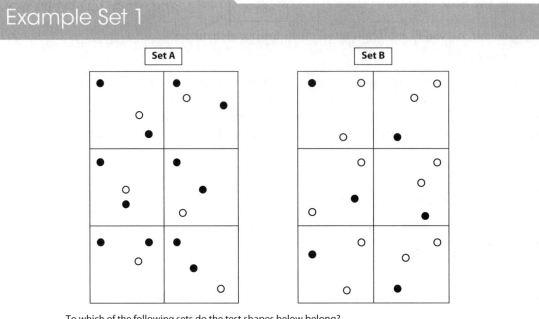

To which of the following sets do the test shapes below belong?

Test Shapes:

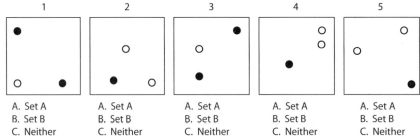

1	2	3	4	5
A. Set A B. Set B C. Neither	A. Set A B. Set B C. Neither	A. Set A B. Set B C. Neither	A. Set A B. Set B C. Neither	A. Set A B. Set B C. Neither

Example Set 1: Answers and Explanations

In this set there are two patterns: position and shading. Both are 'big picture' patterns and easier to see the farther away from the sets you are. In Set A, there are two shaded circles and one unshaded circle in every box, with one shaded circle in the top left-hand corner. In Set B, there are two unshaded circles and one shaded circle in each box, with one unshaded circle in the top right-hand corner.

Test Shape 1: Set A – There are two shaded circles and one unshaded circle, with one shaded circle in the top left-hand corner.

Test Shape 2: Neither – Although it has two unshaded circles and one shaded circle, there is no unshaded circle in the top right-hand corner.

Test Shape 3: Neither – It has the colour distribution for Set A but the position (albeit the wrong shading) for Set B.

Test Shape 4: Set B – There are two unshaded circles, one of which is in the top right-hand corner, and one shaded circle.

Test Shape 5: Set B – Same as above.

Top Tip: If there is more than one pattern present, the question will usually be designed in such a way that spotting one pattern will still score you some points.

Impression 1: Everything Looks the Same

Sometimes you are faced with two sets that look almost identical. There are relatively few patterns that commonly fit this scenario. This is due to the fact that many patterns will cancel themselves out when the two sets use the same item number and type in each box. The main patterns to look for when everything looks the same are:

- Position
- Shading
- Conditional

If you failed to spot both patterns in this example, then look back now. Hopefully you will find it a lot easier now that you know what to look for. Try to apply this in future when faced with near-identical looking sets.

Refer to **Example Set 2** below. Set a timer for 70 seconds and make a note of your answers before moving on to the explanations.

Example Set 2

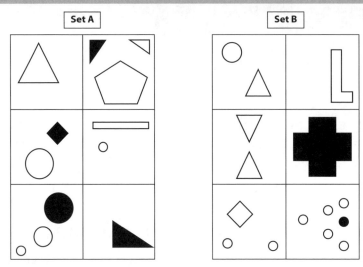

To which of the following sets do the test shapes below belong?

Test Shapes:

| 1 | 2 | 3 | 4 | 5 |

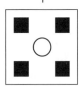 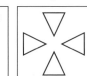 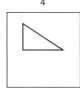

1	2	3	4	5
A. Set A	A. Set A	A. Set A	A. Set A	A. Set A
B. Set B	B. Set B	B. Set B	B. Set B	B. Set B
C. Neither	C. Neither	C. Neither	C. Neither	C. Neither

Example Set 2: Answers and Explanations

There is only one pattern in this set: the total number of sides in every box. In Set A, the total number of sides is an odd number. In Set B, it is an even number. Remember that a circle has one side (not an infinite number of sides, as so many students mistakenly assume). In this case, there is no pattern in terms of shading. The shading merely acts as a distractor.

Top Tip: If you only identify an odd/even pattern then it's important that you look for a second pattern. Otherwise 'Neither' will rarely be a viable answer option.

Test Shape 1: Set A – 17 sides in total

Test Shape 2: Set B – 8 sides in total

Test Shape 3: Set B – 12 sides in total

Test Shape 4: Set A – 3 sides in total

Test Shape 5: Set A – 1 side in total

Impression 2: Different Blocks of Shapes

Seeing boxes comprising seemingly random blocks of shapes can be daunting. It's difficult to know where to begin. Unfortunately, sets consisting of different shapes do lend themselves to numerous potential patterns. There are seven patterns to look for in this situation. Six are common and one is a rare pattern:

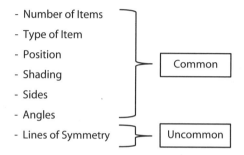

- Number of Items
- Type of Item
- Position
- Shading   Common
- Sides
- Angles
- Lines of Symmetry   Uncommon

The most common angles-based patterns use right angles. If you see right-angled shapes in every box then it is worth counting the number, looking for an absolute or an odd/even pattern.

Top Tip: When faced with random shapes there are a lot of potential patterns to look for. If you see circles, then you can eliminate 'angles' and 'lines of symmetry'.

Refer to **Example Set 3** below. Set a timer for 70 seconds and make a note of your answers before moving on to the explanations.

Example Set 3

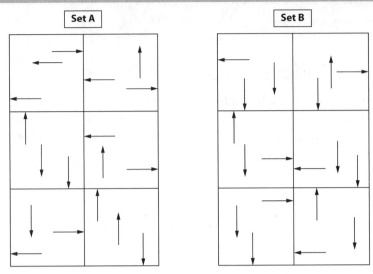

To which of the following sets do the test shapes below belong?

Test Shapes:

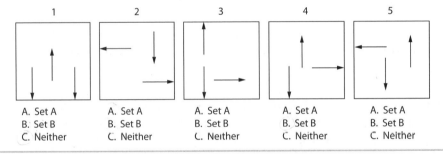

1	2	3	4	5
A. Set A B. Set B C. Neither	A. Set A B. Set B C. Neither	A. Set A B. Set B C. Neither	A. Set A B. Set B C. Neither	A. Set A B. Set B C. Neither

Example Set 3: Answers and Explanations

In these sets all you have is arrows! Each box – in both Set A and Set B – contains three arrows in total, two of which touch the sides. In Set A, the arrows always touch opposite sides. In Set B, however, they touch adjacent sides. There is no other pattern present.

Test Shape 1: Neither – There are two arrows touching sides but they both touch the same side.

Test Shape 2: Set A – There are two arrows touching opposite sides.

Test Shape 3: Set A – There are two arrows touching opposite sides.

Test Shape 4: Set B – There are two arrows touching adjacent sides.

Test Shape 5: Neither – There is only one arrow touching a side.

Impression 3: Arrows by Themselves

Doing an Abstract Reasoning question based entirely on arrows can be overwhelming. The reality is that there is actually quite a limited number of potential patterns that could be present. If all you see are arrows, then the four main patterns to look out for are:

- Number
- Direction
- Position
- Touching sides

Special Circumstances: Touching Sides

It is unusual for shapes to touch the sides of the boxes in abstract reasoning. If you see shapes consistently touching sides then always assess this before looking for other patterns. When items touch sides, there are several possible patterns, depending on:

- Which side(s) is being touched
- The number of sides being touched

Refer to **Example Set 4** below. Set a timer for 70 seconds and make a note of your answers before moving on to the explanations.

Example Set 4

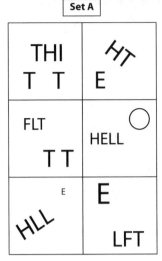

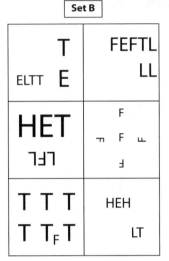

To which of the following sets do the test shapes below belong?

Test Shapes:

1	2	3	4	5

A. Set A
B. Set B
C. Neither

A. Set A
B. Set B
C. Neither

A. Set A
B. Set B
C. Neither

A. Set A
B. Set B
C. Neither

A. Set A
B. Set B
C. Neither

Example Set 4: Answers and Explanations

When seeing a set of questions consisting of words and letters, it is important to remember that these are, in fact, not words and letters per se. Instead, you should view them simply as abstract shapes (that just happen to resemble words and letters). Abstract reasoning is assessing your ability to identify physical patterns. So, any meaning attributed to the shapes does not contribute towards the pattern. In this example, there is only one pattern present: there are 10 right angles per box in Set A and 15 right angles per box in set B. The capital letters E, F, H, L and T are all made up of right angles (E = 4, F = 3, H = 4, L = 1 and T = 2).

Test Shape 1: Set A – 10 right angles

Test Shape 2: Neither – 12 right angles

Test Shape 3: Neither – 16 right angles

Test Shape 4: Set B – 15 right angles

Test Shape 5: Set A – 10 right angles

Impression 4: Letters and Words

Although they look complex, questions involving letters or words are still only assessing the **physical properties** of the 'shapes'. The patterns never relate to meaning. Certain letters (E, F, H, L and T) lend themselves to right angles. So when these letters are present, you must always consider this pattern first. The patterns you should look for when presented with letters and words are:

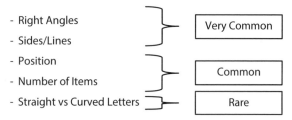

As you are only assessing the physical properties of the shapes – and not the meaning – you should not consider the following as part of a pattern:

- Upper vs lower case
- Vowel vs consonant
- Meanings of the words

Refer to **Example Set 5** below. Set a timer for 70 seconds and make a note of your answers before moving on to the explanations.

Example Set 5

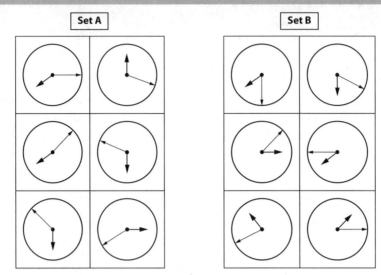

To which of the following sets do the test shapes below belong?

Test Shapes:

1	2	3	4	5

A. Set A B. Set B C. Neither	A. Set A B. Set B C. Neither	A. Set A B. Set B C. Neither	A. Set A B. Set B C. Neither	A. Set A B. Set B C. Neither

Example Set 5: Answers and Explanations

The picture set presents you with a series of 'clocks'. Although, as with all abstract reasoning, they are not truly clocks. Rather, they are combinations of shapes that resemble clocks! The most striking feature you will notice when faced with clock faces are the angles. Although angles are likely to play a part, don't forget to assess the shapes for other physical properties. In this case, both sets contain a large circle, within which there is a long, thin arrow that connects with the circle and a short, fat arrow that does not. In Set A, the angle between the two arrows is obtuse (>90°). In Set B, the angle between the two arrows is acute (<90°).

Test Shape 1: Set B – There is an acute angle between the arrows.

Test Shape 2: Neither – There is a right angle between the arrows, so as a result the angle is neither acute nor obtuse between the arrows.

> Test Shape 3: Set A – There is an obtuse angle between the arrows.
>
> Test Shape 4: Neither – There is an obtuse angle between the arrows, so the test shape initially appears to belong to Set A. However, the long thin arrow does not connect with the circle, and therefore the physical properties are different.
>
> Test Shape 5: Set A – There is an obtuse angle between the arrows.

Impression 5: Familiar Objects

The objects in Set A and Set B may mimic 'familiar' objects, such as clocks, dominoes, or even faces. But they must nevertheless be assessed on the basis of their **physical properties**. The more familiar the object, the easier it is to overlook this crucial point. In the previous example, it is easy to make a mistake on Test Shape 4, where the angle fits with Set A but physical properties differ.

'Clocks' can be presented both as analogue and digital displays. It is crucial to remember that 'time' itself cannot be a pattern. So, having morning vs. evening, for instance, would never work.

Example of a digital clock display:

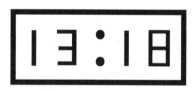

Although the time itself cannot be a pattern, different times will generate different potential patterns. This might include the number of lines or, in the image above, the number of right angles.

Refer to **Example Set 6** below. Set a timer for 70 seconds and make a note of your answers before moving on to the explanations.

Example Set 6

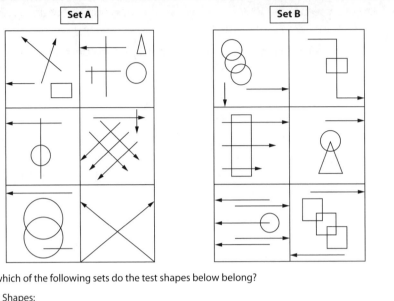

To which of the following sets do the test shapes below belong?

Test Shapes:

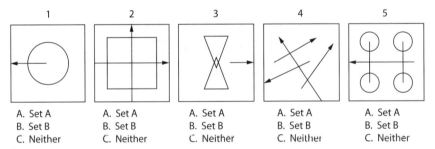

1	2	3	4	5
A. Set A	A. Set A	A. Set A	A. Set A	A. Set A
B. Set B	B. Set B	B. Set B	B. Set B	B. Set B
C. Neither	C. Neither	C. Neither	C. Neither	C. Neither

Example Set 6: Answers and Explanations

In this question set there are two patterns: intersections and touching sides. In Set A, there is an odd number of intersections. But remember: whenever faced with an odd/even pattern you must always look for a second pattern. In this case, there is also an arrow touching the left side of every box. In Set B, there are an even number of intersections and an arrow touching the right side of every box. Touching sides is an unusual pattern, so whenever you see shapes or objects touching the side of the box, always explore this for a pattern (even if other patterns appear obvious).

Test Shape 1: Set A – There is an odd number of intersections and an arrow touching the left.

Test Shape 2: Neither – There is an odd number of intersections but no arrow touching the left.

> Test Shape 3: Set B – There is an even number of intersections and an arrow touching the right.
>
> Test Shape 4: Set A – There is an odd number of intersections and an arrow touching the left.
>
> Test Shape 5: Neither – There is an even number of intersections but no arrow touching the right.

Impression 6: Abstract Patterns

When faced with the apparent randomness of anything from shapes, lines and arrows, to 'squiggly lines', you must always consider:

- Number of items
- Intersections
- Touching sides
- Angles
- Areas

Special Circumstances: Items Overlapping

It is unusual for items to be placed on top of each other. If they are, this creates crossing points known as intersections. Whenever you see this occurring, consider whether this is your underlying pattern.

> **Top Tip:** The point at which a shape touches the side of a box is not an intersection, as technically it does not cross over. So, do not count 'touching sides' as intersections.

Refer to **Example Set 7** below. Set a timer for 70 seconds and make a note of your answers before moving on to the explanations.

Example Set 7

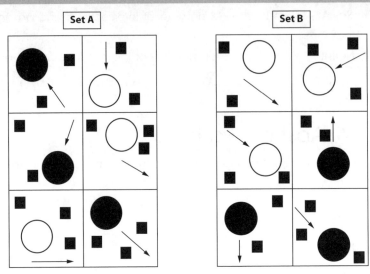

To which of the following sets do the test shapes below belong?

Test Shapes:

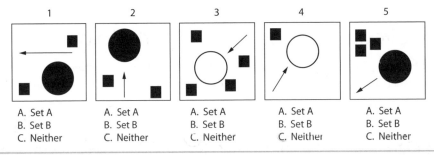

1	2	3	4	5
A. Set A	A. Set A	A. Set A	A. Set A	A. Set A
B. Set B	B. Set B	B. Set B	B. Set B	B. Set B
C. Neither	C. Neither	C. Neither	C. Neither	C. Neither

Example Set 7: Answers and Explanations

This is our first example of a conditional pattern. These occur when the patterns are linked and dependent upon each other. When dealing with conditional patterns, ask yourself: 'If X happens to Y, what happens to Z?' In the above set, you can see that there are arrows either pointing toward the circle or away from it. So, the question is: What happens when the arrow points toward/away from the circle? In Set A, when the arrow points towards the circle there are two squares in each box; when it points away, there are three squares. In Set B, when the arrow points towards the circle there are three squares in each box; when the arrow points away, there are two squares. There is no pattern relating to the position of the squares or shading of the circle.

Test Shape 1: Set B – The arrow points away from the circle and there are two squares.

Test Shape 2: Set A – The arrow points towards the circle and there are two squares.

Test Shape 3: Neither – There are four squares in the test box, which doesn't fit with Set A or B.

Test Shape 4: Neither – There is only one square in the test box, which doesn't fit with the pattern in either Set A or B.

Test Shape 5: Set A – The arrow points away from the circle and there are three squares in the box.

Impression 7: Something's Changing

You look at Set A and Set B. They appear to be very similar. Yet something seems to keep changing. In that case, it's almost certainly a conditional question. Conditional patterns are linked and dependent on each other. In this case, you need to look at the boxes in detail and ascertain which components are changing and how. By doing so, you can figure out the conditional pattern. The five things that are most likely to change in conditional questions are:

- Number of items
- Position
- Shading
- Size of items
- Direction

Special Circumstances: Arrows Pointing to/from Items

If you encounter a question set containing arrows which point either to or from items then this is almost certainly a conditional question. So, your next task is to identify what other patterns arise when direction of the arrow changes.

Refer to **Example Set 8** below. Set a timer for 70 seconds and make a note of your answers before moving on to the explanations.

Example Set 8

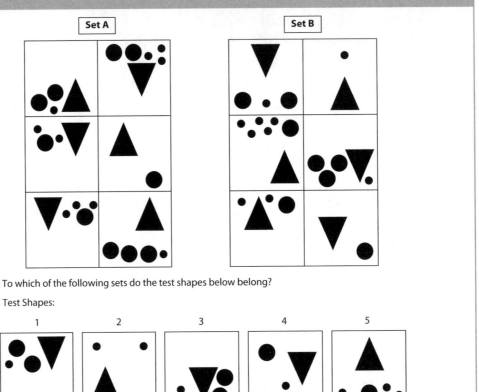

To which of the following sets do the test shapes below belong?

Test Shapes:

1	2	3	4	5
A. Set A B. Set B C. Neither	A. Set A B. Set B C. Neither	A. Set A B. Set B C. Neither	A. Set A B. Set B C. Neither	A. Set A B. Set B C. Neither

Example Set 8: Answers and Explanations

This is another example of a conditional pattern. But this time there are two conditional patterns present: size and position.

In Set A, if the triangle points up, then the circles are in the bottom half of the box and there are more large circles than small ones. If the triangle points down, then the circles are in the top half of the box and there are more small circles than large ones.

The pattern in Set B is the opposite. If the triangle points up, then the circles are in the top half of the box and there are more small circles than large ones. If the triangle points down, then the circles are in the bottom half of the box and there are more large circles than small ones.

Test Shape 1: Neither – The triangle points down and the circles are in the top half. But there are more large circles than small ones. Therefore, the position of the circles is in keeping with Set A, but the size distribution is in keeping with Set B.

Test Shape 2: Set B – The triangle points up and the circles are in the top half of the box, with more small circles than large ones.

Test Shape 3: Set B – The triangle points down and the circles are in the bottom half of the box, with more large circles than small ones.

Test Shape 4: Neither – There are circles in both halves of the box, which is not in keeping with either Set A or B.

Test Shape 5: Neither – The triangle points up and the circles are in the bottom half. But there are more small circles than large ones. Therefore, the position fits with Set A but the size distribution fits with Set B.

Top Tips for Type 1 Questions

1. **Change your perspective** (move closer and further away from the computer screen) to ensure you see both small and big picture patterns.

2. If you can't identify the pattern within **45 seconds** go with your gut instinct, flag the question and **move on**.

3. Always look for **two patterns**, especially if you spot an odd/even distribution, as then there is usually a second pattern also present.

4. Use the **Impression Technique** to quickly narrow down what patterns to look for and what to eliminate.

5. Remember the three **special circumstances**: touching sides, overlapping shapes and arrows pointing to/from items. These rare events often allow you to quickly identify the underlying pattern.

New Question Formats

In 2013, there were three new question styles introduced to the Abstract Reasoning component of the UKCAT exam: Type 2, Type 3 and Type 4.

The Type 2 and 3 questions are 'dynamic' questions. Unlike Type 1 and 4 questions, where you need to identify a fixed pattern and match test shapes accordingly, Type 2 and 3 questions feature a changing pattern. Luckily, students often find it easier to identify this dynamic change, as opposed to static patterns.

Students may have encountered similar question styles to Type 2 and 3 questions in the past. They are a staple of many IQ and career aptitude tests.

Type 2 Questions

In Type 2 questions, you are presented with a series of four boxes of shapes. Changes occur from one box to the next. Your task is to identify what, exactly, is changing and to decide which of four options would come next in the sequence. The time pressure with this question type is significant. You have just under 15 seconds per question, so you must stick ruthlessly to your strategy.

Strategy for Type 2 Questions

1. Break the items in each box into individual 'components'.

2. Focus on one component at a time, looking at how it changes from one box to the next and paying close attention to:

   - Position
   - Shading
   - Direction/rotation
   - Size

3. As you assess each component in turn, eliminate answer options that don't fit with the next anticipated change.

4. Using this technique, you will eliminate answer options one by one until only the correct answer remains.

Refer to **Example Sets 9 to 11**. Set a timer for **45 seconds** and make a note of your answers before moving on to the explanations.

Example Set 9

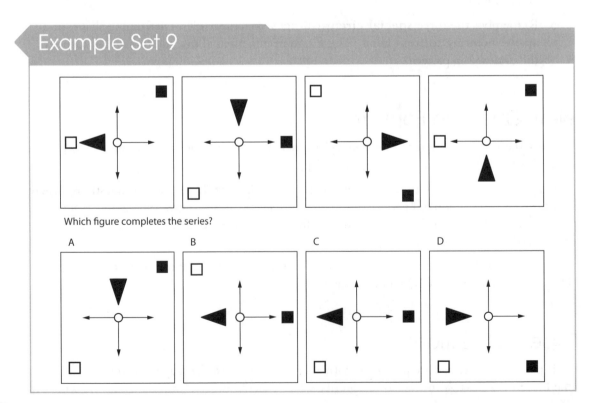

Which figure completes the series?

A   B   C   D

Example Set 10

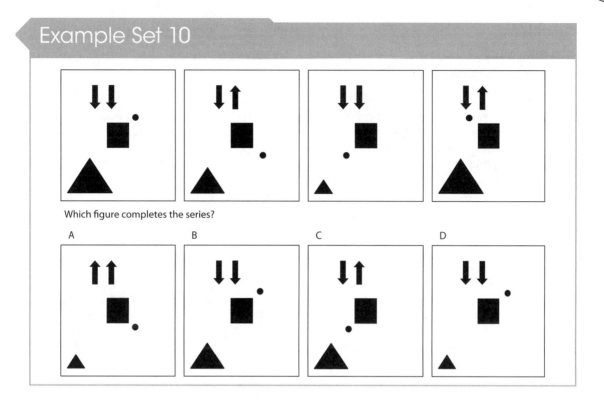

Which figure completes the series?

A   B   C   D

Example Set 11

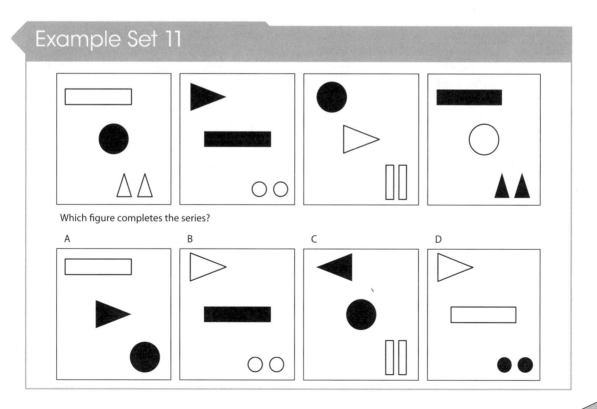

Which figure completes the series?

A   B   C   D

Example Sets 9 to 11: Answers and Explanations

Set 9 – Option C

There are four components to this shape: a central three pronged spoke, a triangle, a black square and a white square. The central spoke rotates clockwise 90° between each box. So, this allows you to eliminate option A. The triangle alternates between pointing toward the spoke and away from it. So, you can also eliminate options A and D. Both the black square and white square move in the same way between the boxes: from the top, to the middle, to the bottom, then back to the top again. Looking at the white square alone allows you to eliminate option B. Looking at the black square allows you to eliminate A and D. It doesn't matter on which component you begin. But you can often reach the correct answer through elimination, without having to assess every aspect.

Set 10 – Option B

There are many changing elements in this set: a central square with associated black circle, which rotates 90° each time; a triangle in the bottom left corner that changes size from large to medium to small then back to large again; and a combination of two arrows, where the right-hand arrow alternates between pointing down and up, and the left-hand arrow is static and pointing down. Applying these rules allows us to see the only possible answer is B.

Set 11 – Option D

Again, this question features a number of patterns that keep changing. First, the position of the items changes so that the item in the top left corner moves to the middle, then the bottom right-hand corner, before returning to the top left. Second, when the item reaches the bottom right-hand corner, it divides into two identical but smaller copies, which rotate 90° clockwise. The item then returns to its original size and number when moving back into the top left-hand corner. Finally, the shading of each item alternates between shaded and unshaded. After the process of elimination, only answer option D remains.

Type 3 Questions

Like Type 2 questions, Type 3 questions assess your ability to identify a dynamic pattern. You are given two shapes that somehow relate to each other. You will then be given a third shape, and asked which one of four options would, by the same logic, relate to that. The time pressure is once again intense, with just under 15 seconds available per question. So, strategy and stamina are essential.

Strategy for Type 3 Questions

The strategy employed for Type 3 questions is similar to that used for Type 2:

1. Focus on the individual components of the example box, one by one.

2. Identify which components have changed and which have remained static.

3. These static components must also remain static in your new test box.

4. Identify and apply the dynamic changes to your test shape, eliminating answers options that don't match until you are left with the correct answer.

Refer to **Example Sets 12 and 13** below. Set a timer for **30 seconds** and make a note of your answers before moving on to the explanations.

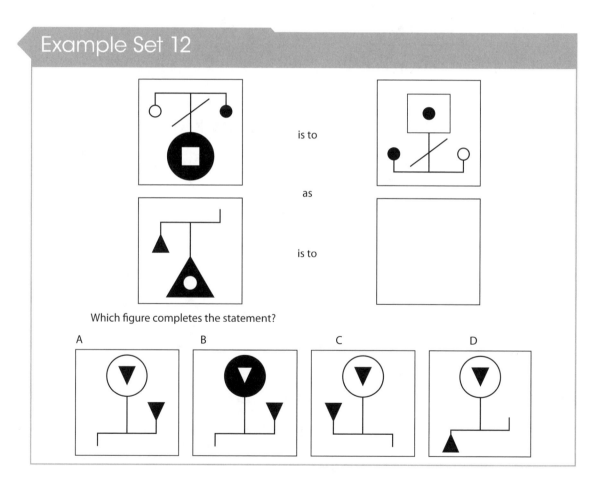

Example Set 12

Which figure completes the statement?

A   B   C   D

Example Set 13

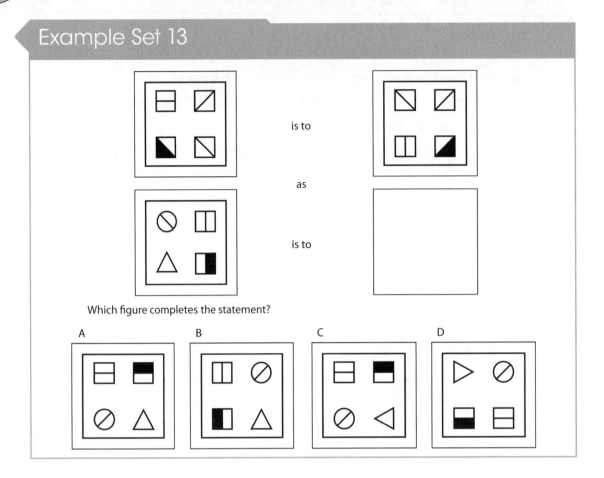

is to

as

is to

Which figure completes the statement?

A   B   C   D

Example Sets 12 and 13: Answers and Explanations

Set 12 – Option A

Rotation and direction are particularly important in Type 3 questions. Looking at the demonstration set shows you that the entire structure rotates 180° clockwise. You can quickly deduce this, as the position of the shaded and unshaded circles swaps around, while the intersecting straight line remains upward sloping. If it had inverted, then the position of the shaded and unshaded circles would have remained the same, while the angle of the intersecting straight line would have become downward sloping. The second change is that the circle and square swap size and position (but not shading).

When you apply these rules to your test shape, you will see that Option A fits the above rules. In Option B, the circle and triangle have swapped shading as well as size and position, which is incorrect. Option C would fit with inversion, not rotation. And Option D is not viable, as the triangle has moved to the outside of the structure.

Set 13 – Option C

This kind of combination of shapes can be quite confusing at first. But if you look at the structure contained within the square as a whole, you will notice that the only change is that the entire structure has rotated 90° anti-clockwise. There are no further changes taking place to any of the smaller shapes within the square.

In Option A, the problem lies with the triangle: the direction is wrong. If the triangle had rotated 90° anti-clockwise, it would point towards the circle – as in the correct answer, Option C. Option B is incorrect as it is the result of a side-to-side inversion. In Option D, the whole structure has rotated 90° clockwise instead of anti-clockwise.

Type 4 Questions

Type 4 questions are, in essence, almost identical to Type 1. They are just more time pressured! You will be presented with two sets of shapes: Set A and Set B. This time, however, you do not get a series of test shapes to match to one set or another. Instead, you are presented with four test shapes simultaneously and asked one of two questions:

- Which of the following test shapes belongs in Set A?

  OR

- Which of the following test shapes belongs in Set B?

So, you need to utilise precisely the same skills employed when answering Type 1 questions, in order to identify the pattern in Set A and Set B. This will allow you to answer either of the questions posed above.

Time for some practice! Try answering the following **11 Practice Sets** containing **55 questions**. There is a mixture of Type 1, 2, 3 and 4 questions. You have 13 minutes to answer all questions. Detailed explanations are provided. Good luck!

Practice Sets

Question Set 1

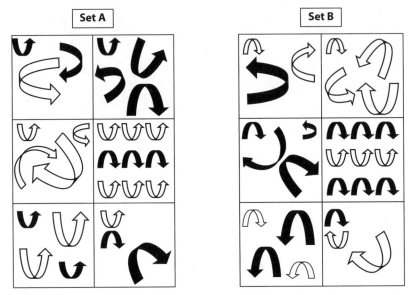

To which of the following sets do the test shapes below belong?

Test Shapes:

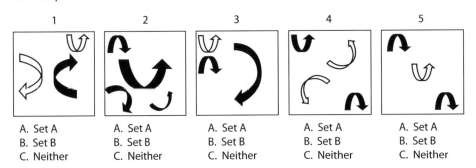

1	2	3	4	5
A. Set A	A. Set A	A. Set A	A. Set A	A. Set A
B. Set B	B. Set B	B. Set B	B. Set B	B. Set B
C. Neither	C. Neither	C. Neither	C. Neither	C. Neither

Question Set 2

Set A

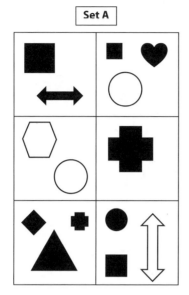

Set B

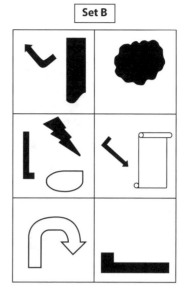

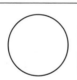   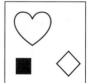

To which of the following sets do the test shapes below belong?

Test Shapes:

1	2	3	4	5

A. Set A   A. Set A   A. Set A   A. Set A   A. Set A
B. Set B   B. Set B   B. Set B   B. Set B   B. Set B
C. Neither   C. Neither   C. Neither   C. Neither   C. Neither

Question Set 3

Set A

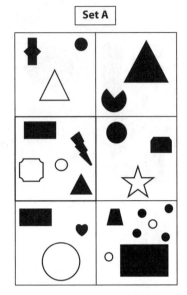

Set B

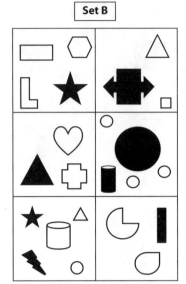

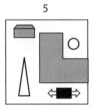

To which of the following sets do the test shapes below belong?

Test Shapes:

1	2	3	4	5

1

A. Set A
B. Set B
C. Neither

2

A. Set A
B. Set B
C. Neither

3

A. Set A
B. Set B
C. Neither

4

A. Set A
B. Set B
C. Neither

5

A. Set A
B. Set B
C. Neither

Question Set 4

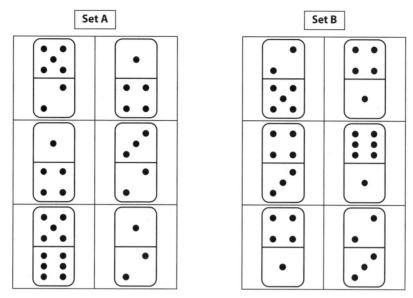

To which of the following sets do the test shapes below belong?

Test Shapes:

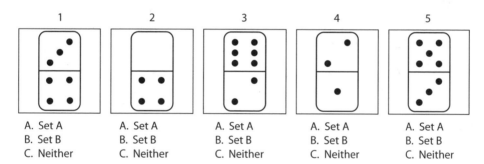

1	2	3	4	5
A. Set A	A. Set A	A. Set A	A. Set A	A. Set A
B. Set B	B. Set B	B. Set B	B. Set B	B. Set B
C. Neither	C. Neither	C. Neither	C. Neither	C. Neither

Question Set 5

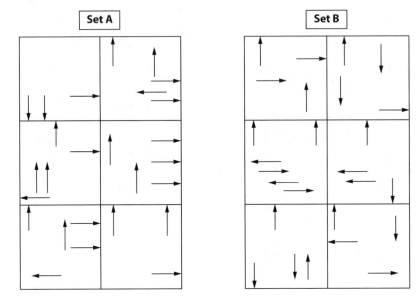

To which of the following sets do the test shapes below belong?

Test Shapes:

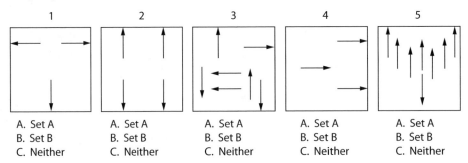

1	2	3	4	5
A. Set A	A. Set A	A. Set A	A. Set A	A. Set A
B. Set B	B. Set B	B. Set B	B. Set B	B. Set B
C. Neither	C. Neither	C. Neither	C. Neither	C. Neither

Question Set 6

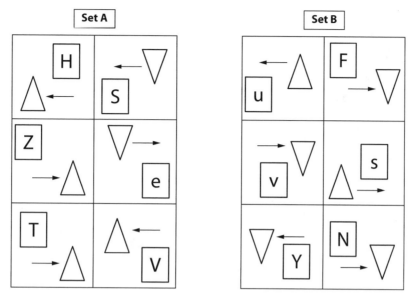

To which of the following sets do the test shapes below belong?

Test Shapes:

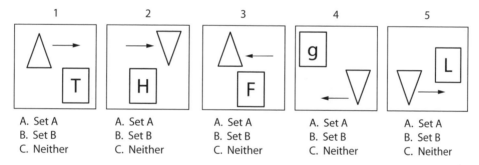

A. Set A
B. Set B
C. Neither

A. Set A
B. Set B
C. Neither

A. Set A
B. Set B
C. Neither

A. Set A
B. Set B
C. Neither

A. Set A
B. Set B
C. Neither

Question Set 7

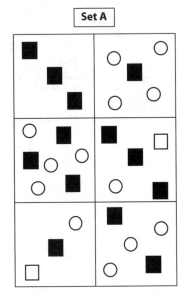

Set A

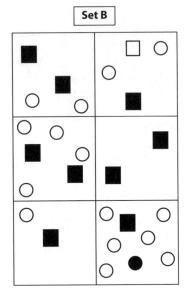

Set B

To which of the following sets do the test shapes below belong?

Test Shapes:

1	2	3	4	5
A. Set A	A. Set A	A. Set A	A. Set A	A. Set A
B. Set B	B. Set B	B. Set B	B. Set B	B. Set B
C. Neither	C. Neither	C. Neither	C. Neither	C. Neither

Question Set 8

Set A

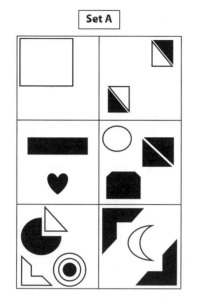

Set B

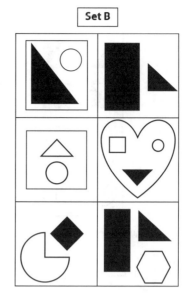

To which of the following sets do the test shapes below belong?

Test Shapes:

1	2	3	4	5

A. Set A	A. Set A	A. Set A	A. Set A	A. Set A
B. Set B	B. Set B	B. Set B	B. Set B	B. Set B
C. Neither	C. Neither	C. Neither	C. Neither	C. Neither

Question Set 9

Question 1

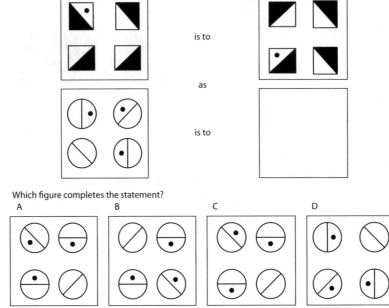

Which figure completes the statement?

A   B   C   D

Question 2

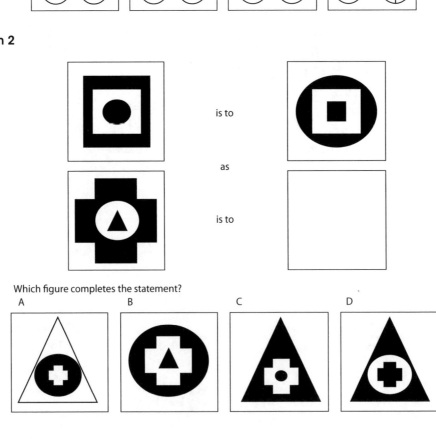

Which figure completes the statement?

A   B   C   D

Question 3

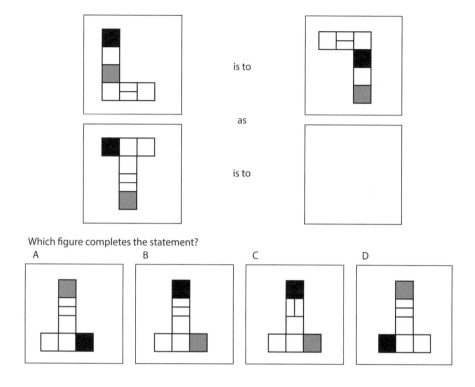

Which figure completes the statement?

A B C D

Question 4

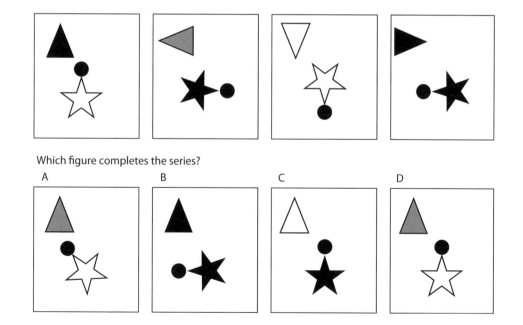

Which figure completes the series?

A B C D

Question 5

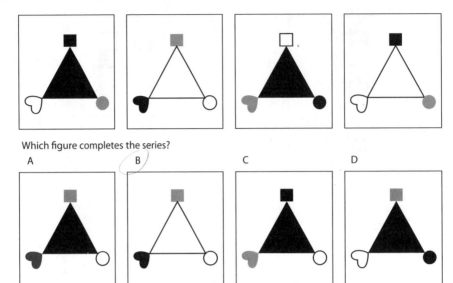

Which figure completes the series?

A   B   C   D

Question Set 10

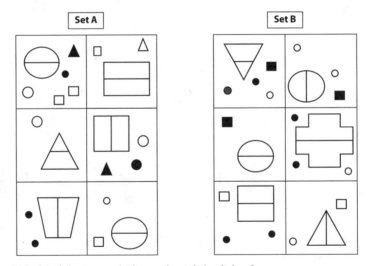

To which of the following sets do the test shapes below belong?

Test Shapes:

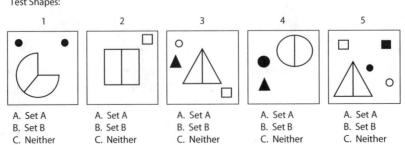

1	2	3	4	5
A. Set A	A. Set A	A. Set A	A. Set A	A. Set A
B. Set B	B. Set B	B. Set B	B. Set B	B. Set B
C. Neither	C. Neither	C. Neither	C. Neither	C. Neither

Question Set 11

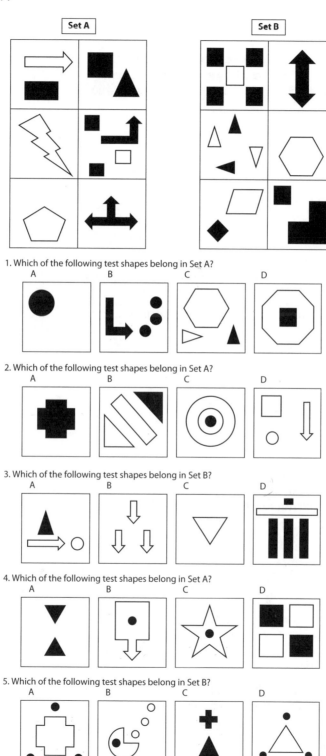

1. Which of the following test shapes belong in Set A?
   A   B   C   D

2. Which of the following test shapes belong in Set A?
   A   B   C   D

3. Which of the following test shapes belong in Set B?
   A   B   C   D

4. Which of the following test shapes belong in Set A?
   A   B   C   D

5. Which of the following test shapes belong in Set B?
   A   B   C   D

Answers

Question Set 1

This question is relatively straight forward and is looking at the position of objects. In Set A there is an upward facing curved arrow in the top left corner of each box, while in set B there is a downward facing curved arrow in the top left corner of each box.

Test Shape 1: Neither

Test Shape 2: Set B

Test Shape 3: Set A

Test Shape 4: Set A

Test Shape 5: Set B

Question Set 2

This question is quite tricky but again is only testing one theme: symmetry. In Set A all the shapes are symmetrical, whereas in Set B they are not.

Test Shape 1: Neither (as it is a mix of symmetrical and non-symmetrical shapes)

Test Shape 2: Set A

Test Shape 3: Set B

Test Shape 4: Set B

Test Shape 5: Set A

Question Set 3

This question set contains boxes that contain seemingly similar shapes with no obvious pattern. The pattern present is that in Set A there are always more shaded than non-shaded shapes in each box, with the reverse true for Set B.

Test Shape 1: Set A

Test Shape 2: Set A

Test Shape 3: Neither

Test Shape 4: Set B

Test Shape 5: Set B

Question Set 4

In this question you are faced with dominoes, but again remember to treat them as shapes and look for the same types of pattern as you would normally. In Set A there is an odd number on top with an even number below, with the reverse pattern in set B.

Test Shape 1: Set A

Test Shape 2: Neither

Test Shape 3: Neither

Test Shape 4: Set B

Test Shape 5: Neither

Question Set 5

This question is hard as it is looking at various themes simultaneously. In Set A, there are always an odd number of arrows in total, with three arrows touching sides in every box and an arrow touching the right-hand side of the box in every shape. In Set B there are an even total number of arrows, an arrow touching the top side of each box and a total of two arrows touching sides in each box.

Test Shape 1: Set A

Test Shape 2: Neither

Test Shape 3: Set A

Test Shape 4: Neither

Test Shape 5: Set B

Question Set 6

This question is difficult. There are several themes to spot, including a conditional theme. In Set A, when a triangle faces up, there is an arrow pointing towards the triangle as well as a box containing a letter made up of straight lines only. When the triangle faces down, the arrow faces away from the triangle and the letter in the box is curved. In Set B, when a triangle faces up, there is an arrow pointing away from the triangle and the letter in the box is curved, while, when the triangle points down, the arrow points towards the triangle and the letter in the box is made up of straight lines.

Test Shape 1: Neither (to fit into Set A the arrow should face towards the triangle)

Test Shape 2: Set B

Test Shape 3: Set A

Test Shape 4: Set A

Test Shape 5: Neither

Question Set 7

All the boxes look very similar, but the only pattern present is that in Set A there is an odd number of shapes in each box, whereas in Set B there is an even number.

Test Shape 1: Set A

Test Shape 2: Set B

Test Shape 3: Set A

Test Shape 4: Set A

Test Shape 5: Set B

Question Set 8

This question is looking at the number of right angles. In Set A there are four right angles in each box, whereas in Set B there are five in each box.

Test Shape 1: Neither

Test Shape 2: Set A

Test Shape 3: Neither

Test Shape 4: Set B

Test Shape 5: Set B

Question Set 9

Question 1 – Option A

This is an example of a Type 3 question presenting you with a 'statement' between two shapes. If you consider the four squares together as a collective, then the combined 'macro structure' rotates 90° anti-clockwise between the two shapes. If you apply the same rules, considering the four circles in the test shape as one large structure and rotating it 90° anti-clockwise, you will get Option A.

Question 2 – Option D

In the demonstration shapes of this Type 3 question there are three objects: two squares and a circle. The object changes in such a way that the inside and outside shapes swap place (and size) so that the circle that was on the inside is now on the outside and the black square that was on the outside is now on the inside. The middle square remains unchanged. If you apply the same changes to the test shape the resulting new shape is Option D.

Question 3 – Option B

This is another example of a Type 3 question. The demonstration shape is rotated 180° between the two boxes, which allows you to eliminate answer option C as the line within one of the boxes is orientated in the wrong direction. The next, and only other change, is that the two shaded boxes swap places. As such the black box appears where the grey box was and vice versa. If you apply the same rules to your test shape only option B fits.

Question 4 – Option D

This is a Type 2 question where you must find the next shape in the sequence. There are four items changing between each step: the triangle rotates 90° anti-clockwise between each step, the triangle changes colour from black to grey to white then back to black again, the star changes colour alternating between white and black and the star with the attached circle rotates 90° clockwise each time (note the difference between the whole structure rotating 90° clockwise and the circle moving from one tip to the next). When you apply the above rules the triangle should point up and be grey, while the star should have the circle at the top (as it would have completed a full 360° rotation) and be coloured white. Only option D fits this description.

Question 5 – Option A

This is another Type 2 question where the main change from one box to the next is colour. The small shapes change colour from black to grey to white then back to black again, while the triangle simply alternates between black and white. There is no change in position or type of item. Following these rules, the next shape should contain a black triangle in the centre with the small shapes containing a grey square, black heart and white circle: option A.

Question Set 10

Question 10 is a Type 1 question with a conditional pattern. In Set A if the large shape has a horizontal line there are more unshaded than shaded small shapes, whereas if the large shape has a vertical line there are more shaded than unshaded small shapes. The reverse is true in Set B where if there is a horizontal line there are more shaded than unshaded small shapes, while if the large shape has a vertical line there are more unshaded than shaded small shapes.

> Test Shape 1: Neither (as there is neither a vertical nor horizontal line)
>
> Test Shape 2: Set B
>
> Test Shape 3: Set B
>
> Test Shape 4: Set A
>
> Test Shape 5: Neither (as there are an equal number of shaded and unshaded small shapes)

Question Set 11

This is a Type 4 question. In Set A there are an odd number of total sides within each box, while in Set B there is an even number of total sides. There is no other pattern present but, as there are more shapes to evaluate for each question, the Type 4 questions are more time consuming than type 1 questions, despite being almost identical in most other respects. It is very important to make sure you read each question carefully to ensure you are looking for the correct test shape.

> Question 1: Option A (1 side, odd)
>
> Question 2: Option C (3 sides, odd)
>
> Question 3: Option D (20 sides, even)
>
> Question 4: Option C (11 sides, odd)
>
> Question 5: Option D (6 sides, even)

CHAPTER 4

Decision Analysis

Overview

The Decision Analysis (DA) section of the UKCAT represents a shift away from pure logical reasoning into a 'grey area', where you are required to make a judgement call to select the best fitting answer. In 2013 this was the highest scoring section, with candidates scoring an average of 771 points – over 200 points higher than the verbal reasoning section. The UKCAT board has, however, made this section more difficult, and in 2014, students found the questions much more challenging. This was reflected by the average score falling to 614.

Format of the Section

You will be faced with 28 questions to be answered in 32 minutes (including 1 minute of reading time). This gives just over 66 seconds per question. In the 2013 sitting this time allowance was generous, with students often finishing in half the time. However, in 2014, many students reported being unable to finish the section in the allocated time.

There are three question styles in decision analysis:

*   Decode and interpret
*   Recode
*   Add new words

The questions are all based around a set of codes. This set of codes consists of a table with letters and numbers correlating to different words. You must use this table to code and decode messages and interpret the meaning.

Codes and Powerful Codes

The table of codes consists of letters and numbers presented in ascending order, each of which correlates to a different word. Approximately halfway through the section this table expands, roughly doubling the number of codes available and therefore offering more variety for question generation.

Some codes are so-called powerful codes. This is because they can either drastically alter the meaning of words they are subsequently combined with, or they have an effect on the overall meaning or interpretation of the sentence. Let's look at an example.

You have decoded part of a question as 'increase man'. How many new words or phrases can you think of that might represent a fair interpretation of 'increase man'?

'Increase' could be taken to mean a number of different things. It could refer to number, thereby changing the phrase 'increase man' to 'men'. Maybe 'increase' refers to size, in which case 'tall man' and 'fat man' could both conceivably be options. It could also refer to a characteristic such as age, creating 'old man'. If you think outside the box, then maybe 'increase' could mean increase in the sense of social status, creating 'king'. Or maybe 'increase man' could mean a more manly man or a muscular man. Ultimately, there will always be numerous ways to interpret the combination of codes with powerful codes.

Commonly Encountered Powerful Codes			
Increase	Decrease	Forward	Reverse
Add	Remove	Generalise	Personalise
Positive	Negative	Past	Future
Plural	Opposite	Command	Emotion

Although this list is not exhaustive, you can easily see how these commonly occurring powerful codes can drastically change the meaning of words with which they are combined, as well as affect the sentence as a whole (such as using 'past' or 'future' to change tense).

> **Top Tip:** Always think 'outside the box' and don't simply take translations as their pure literal meaning.

Basic Rules and Principles

The codes you are presented with will be broken up into bite-sized sections using commas and brackets. Commas are used to separate sections of the code, but the order of these sections is irrelevant. The first section could, for instance, code for the last part of the sentence.

Codes that are grouped together by brackets, however, follow stricter rules. Anything contained within the brackets must remain grouped together and cannot be combined with codes elsewhere in the sentence. In other words, brackets follow the same rules they do in mathematics.

Decision Analysis Layout

The computer screenshot of the decision analysis section is slightly different to that of the other sections. The information area on the left-hand side of the screen now contains four tabs which you can scroll through. The tabs are:

- **Passage:** This is a fictional short story designed to place your code into context of how it was discovered or might have been used. Often this involves you exploring old houses or pyramids, or stumbling across long-lost codes you must 'decipher'. Ultimately it has no bearing on the code itself or how you answer questions, but it will use up your valuable time!

- **Example 1 and Example 2:** These are two worked examples where you are given a code with five potential answers and told which one is correct. It is designed to allow you to work out how the code functions and apply the same rules going forward when you encounter the same codes in your questions.

- **Table of codes:** This is the most important tab as it contains the table of codes you require to solve the questions. You should keep this tab open at all times when answering questions.

Confidence Rating Trial

In 2013 and again in 2014 the UKCAT board conducted a trial of a confidence rating system. After each question in the Decision Analysis section students had to rate how confident they were that the answer they gave was correct on a scale of 1–5, with 1 being 'not confident at all' and 5 being 'very confident'. In 2013 and 2014 this rating had no impact on your score and was not communicated to your university; it was for internal use only. Students were, however, forced to participate in the trial and couldn't move on from one question to the next without submitting a confidence rating score.

The confidence rating trial shows that the UKCAT board are considering the introduction of negatively marked questions. Confidence rating only works if there are negatively marked questions, as there has to be a risk as well as a reward. Typically these systems score you more marks the more confident you are and penalise you heavily if you are very confident but wrong. Whether or not a formal confidence scoring system or negatively marked questions will be introduced for the 2015 sitting remains to be seen.

Decode and Interpret Questions

The 'decode and interpret' style questions make up approximately two-thirds of the Decision Analysis section. You are presented with a code followed by five potential translations. Your task is to use your best judgement to select which of the five options you feel is the best interpretation of the code.

The problem with decision analysis is that there is no one perfect logical answer. In 2013 the DA questions were relatively straightforward, with relatively little ambiguity and only one or two viable answer options per question. In 2014, however, many students found they were only able to narrow the five options down to two or three viable answers, after which they struggled to select between them. It is therefore essential to have a strategy to effectively eliminate options and settle on the correct answer.

Strategy for Decode and Interpret Questions

1. Ignore the introductory passage

   The introductory passage is simply a fairy tale and, although often interesting, it does not add any value to you, nor does it help you answer any subsequent questions. It does, however, consume your time!

2. Quickly scan the worked examples

The two tabs, Example 1 and Example 2, provide you with two sample questions where they tell you the correct answer. It is your opportunity to see how some of the powerful operators work and then apply these rules going forward in subsequent questions. It is, however, important not to spend too much time on this section; otherwise you will find yourself struggling to finish.

3. Write out the full translation of the code for each question

In order to improve your chances of successfully decoding the question we recommend writing out the full literal translation of the code into your laminated booklet. Keep the commas and brackets as they are but substitute the letters and numbers for words. This allows you to easily compare the code to each potential answer without having to remember. This reduces the chance of making a mistake, especially when dealing with longer or trickier codes. With the trend in 2014 being towards having more ambiguity in the answers, this technique becomes essential.

4. Eliminate answer options

Once you have the full translation of the code you must analyse each answer option in turn, eliminating incorrect ones and leaving the correct answer. As you work through the chapter you will learn what to look for and how to eliminate potential answer options.

We will now work our way through numerous examples, looking at how to eliminate answer options.

Refer to **Example Set 1** below. Set a timer for 330 seconds (5.5 minutes) and make a note of your answers before moving on to the explanations.

Example Set 1

You are walking down the beach one day when you come across a bottle that has washed up on the shore. Looking inside you find a series of codes and messages written on an old faded sheet of paper. You quickly realise the messages are from the survivors of a ship-wreck. You decide to solve the puzzle to identify what happened.

A	Increase	103	Boy	468	Transport
B	Plural	124	Person	667	Broken
F	Future	177	Money	727	Happy
J	Generalise	223	Boat	741	Little
M	Negative	342	Bicycle	892	Two
P	Personalise	389	Spain	900	Holiday
S	Opposite	443	Hard	904	Cloud

Question 1: A 904, M (P 900)

A. Big clouds cause bad holidays.

B. Storms have given me bad holidays.

C. The storm gave me a bad holiday.

D. A big cloud ruined my holiday in Spain.

E. There are always storms when I go on holiday.

Question 2: A 103, 468, 389, P (741 223)

A. The boys travelled abroad on my small boat.

B. The man travelled to Spain with me on a small boat.

C. The man sailed to Spain on my small boat.

D. My small boat took the tall boys to Spain.

E. The group of boys took a small boat to Spain.

Question 3: F, P (S 727), 667, P 223

A. I will become sad if my boat breaks.

B. I am unhappy because my boat has broken.

C. I am very unhappy as my boat broke.

D. In the future I will be unhappy as my boats will have broken.

E. My broken boats have made me sad.

Question 4: 892 (A 103), J (342 468), B (741 342)

A. The two groups of boys ride small mopeds.

B. Two boys cycled on two small bicycles.

C. Two tall boys rode small mopeds.

D. Two men cycled on small bicycles.

E. Two tall boys cycled on two small bicycles.

Question 5: (B 124), ((S 900) 443, J 177), J (468 389)

A. The people worked hard to earn money to fly to Spain.

B. People work hard to fund travel abroad.

C. The group did not earn enough money to travel to Spain.

D. The group worked hard to go on holiday.

E. Hard working people can fund holidays to Spain.

Example Set 1: Answers and Explanations

Question 1: C. The storm gave me a bad holiday.

The literal translation of the code is: increase cloud, negative (personalise holiday)

- A. There is no representation of the code 'P – personalise' in the answer, making it incomplete. Furthermore, both clouds and holidays are plural here, yet singular in the code (increase cloud could either be big cloud or clouds, but not big clouds as then you would have used increase twice).

- B. Storms is incorrect; although 'increase cloud' could be interpreted as a storm it could not be storms as this would have used increase twice – once to make it big and once to make it plural. 'Holidays' is also incorrect as it should be singular.

- C. Correct

- D. There is an extra word here – 'Spain' – which is not anywhere to be found in the code.

- E. There is an extra word that is not coded for – 'always'. The same issue concerning the plural for storms outlined in option B also applies here.

Question 2: C. The man sailed to Spain on my small boat.

The literal translation of the code is: increase boy, transport, Spain, personalise (little boat)

- A. Although this could be interpreted as being correct, the code '389' codes for Spain and not abroad. It is, therefore, not an ideal translation.

- B. The brackets have been multiplied out incorrectly. 'Personalise' refers to the small boat and must therefore remain combined with the small boat, to make 'my small boat'.

- C. Correct

- D. Although 'took' is not the best translation of transport this might conceivably work. However, when combined with the fact that 'increase boy' has been incorrectly combined into 'the tall boys' ('increase boy' could make 'tall boy' or 'boys' but not 'tall boys', as this uses increase twice) then this makes option D incorrect.

- E. There are numerous errors in this answer. The 'group of boys' has been incorrectly generated from 'increase boy' and there is no representation of 'personalise' any-where in the answer.

Question 3: A. I will become sad if my boat breaks.

The literal translation of the code is: future, personalise (opposite happy), broken, person-alise boat

- A. Correct

- B. The code starts with 'F – future' denoting the fact that there is a tense element to this question. The code is written in the future tense but answer B is in the present tense.

C.   This answer is in the wrong tense and also has the extra word 'very'.

D.   Although the tense is correct there is an error of plurals as boat should be singular and not plural.

E.   There is both an error in tense, as it should be in the future tense, and plurals, as boat should be singular and not plural.

Question 4: D. Two men cycled on small bicycles.

The literal translation of the code is: two (increase boy), generalise (bike transport), plural (little bicycle)

A.   There are a couple of errors in this answer option. First, two groups of boys is a poor translation of 'two (increase boy)'. Second, 'small moped' is incorrect. Although a small bike might conceivably be translated into a moped, the fact that the answer has 'small moped' means that you would have used 'small' twice, thus making it incorrect.

B.   There is no representation of 'increase' in relation to boys in the first part of the sentence. The last part, 'two small bicycles', is more specific than the code, which codes for 'plural (little bikes)' and not a specific number.

C.   This option has the same problem for 'mopeds' as in answer A.

D.   Correct

E.   This would be the second best answer. Although not grossly incorrect, though, it is equally not the best answer option. The last part – 'two small bicycles' – is more specific than the code, which represents 'plural (little bikes)' and not a specific number.

Question 5: B. People work hard to fund travel abroad.

The literal translation of the code is: (plural person), ((opposite holiday) hard, generalise money), generalise (transport Spain)

A.   There is a subtle error here when multiplying out the brackets at the end of the sentence. 'Generalise' needs to multiply into 'transport' and 'Spain' due to the position of the brackets. If you generalise something you make it less specific. Therefore, if you combine 'generalise' with 'Spain', then any answer which still has 'Spain' as an option must be incorrect as you have not generalised it. You can therefore also eliminate answer options C and E.

B.   Correct

C.   This option has introduced a negative into the answer which isn't in the code and also has the same error of incorrectly multiplying out the brackets as in option A.

D.   There is no representation of 'J 177 – generalise money' anywhere in the answer, thereby making it incorrect.

E.   This option has the same error of incorrectly multiplying out the brackets as in option A.

Summary of Common Answer Errors

Although the section is called 'decode and interpret', it is best thought of as 'decode and eliminate'. As you look through the answer options, you're interpreting the best option as the one with no, or fewest, mistakes. By working your way through the example questions above you will have encountered and learnt to recognise the common 'tricks' that make answers incorrect.

Missing Codes:	Some answer options will be incomplete as they do not represent the full code and are missing words.
Extra Codes:	Some answers will have introduced additional words into the answer not represented by the code. In the case of nouns and verbs, these are usually quite obvious. However, adjectives can be very subtle.
Wrong Codes:	Sometimes the answer will have used the wrong translation of the code or inaccurately generated new words by using the powerful operators incorrectly.
Incorrect Brackets:	It is important that you treat brackets just like you would in maths. Codes contained within brackets must remain linked and a code out-side the brackets must be multiplied into the contents of the bracket.
Plurals:	Pay close attention to the number of items specified in the code and how this correlates to the answer. If you have a single item in the code, then answers with plurals are likely to be wrong.
Tense:	Tense is a more ambiguous error. There are codes used that can alter the tense, such as future or past, but these are not always present. If there is no mention of tense in the code then it is unlikely that the tense is relevant. (Although if you can't find any other error then you will have to use tense to narrow your options.)

> **Top Tip:** Use this list of common 'errors' to help you identify which of the options has the fewest, if any, mistakes, thereby identifying the correct answer.

Making Questions Difficult

There are four main ways that the exam writers can make the questions more difficult:

1. Increase the ambiguity

2. Make the codes longer

3. Introduce more brackets

4. Repeat the same code numerous times

By making the codes longer you make the exercise more time pressured. When combining this with an increased use of brackets, there is more scope for making mistakes. Another trick is to repeat the same code several times within one question as it's then easy to overlook how many times you've used it. When questions repeat powerful operators people often go wrong as they feel as if they've already used the code once and overlook further uses. It is vital that, if you see the same code appear more than once in a question, you are meticulous in counting the number of times it appears – both in the question and in your chosen answer – to make sure it matches.

Dealing with Ambiguity

In 2014 the DA was generally found to be more difficult than in previous years, mainly because of increased ambiguity. The questions encountered were not as clear cut as the practice questions previously released. There appeared to be significant overlap and similarities between the answers.

As you work your way through, eliminating potential answer options, there are some errors that clearly will make it impossible for a given option to be correct. However, some of the errors are not quite so clear-cut. To introduce ambiguity, you may find yourself in a situation where all answers appear wrong so you must find the 'least wrong' answer.

There are some 'hard' errors to look out for. Where these are present, the answer option must be wrong. These include:

- Missing codes
- Extra codes
- Wrong codes
- Incorrect brackets

The other two errors – plurals and tense – are not quite so clear cut.

If you go back to Question 4 from Example Set 1, you can see this at work in options B, D and E. The last part of the sentence codes for 'plural (little bicycle)'. The best answer uses the option of 'small bicycles'. However, options B and E have 'two small bicycles'. Technically this is not incorrect – as plural bicycle could be two bicycles. But 'bicycles' would be a better fit as it is less specific: plural but with no absolute value. Plurals are therefore an example of an error which can be both clear cut (for example, if there is a plural in the code but a singular in the answer), or ambiguous (for example, when there is a plural in the question but the answer has an absolute plural value).

Questions may have answer options in different tenses. But unless there is something in the code that denotes tense as being relevant (e.g. codes such as 'future', 'present' or 'past') then you must assume that tense is not relevant. It can, however, be taken into account if you're left in an ambiguous situation where you are struggling to decide between answer options.

There will be 'grey areas' in some of the questions. You should therefore stick to the technique of first eliminating answers with 'hard' errors. After that, you can look at the soft reasons to decide which is the 'least wrong'.

Recode Questions

Recode questions make up approximately a third of the total questions. They are the opposite of the 'decode and interpret' style. You are presented with a sentence and have to choose from among four or five codes the one you feel would best translate into that sentence. All the same rules apply as above, but this time in reverse. For example, some codes will have too many letters or numbers (extra codes), some might have too few (missing codes), and some will have brackets in the wrong place.

Strategy for Recode Questions

1. Focus section by section

   Each of the four or five answer options will be divided up into groups of code, separated by commas and brackets. Begin by looking at the first group in the first answer option.

2. Eliminate groups

   When focusing on each group look out for the same errors as in the 'decode and interpret' section. This includes: missing codes, extra codes, wrong codes, wrongly used brackets, plurals and tenses. If there are no errors, move on to the next group. Once you identify a group that must be incorrect, then you can eliminate this group and that answer option, as well as subsequent answer options that contain the same group.

3. Eliminate answer options

   Every time you can eliminate a group you can eliminate that answer option, as well as subsequent answer options that contain the same group. Keep moving through the options until you are left with one correct answer.

Example Set 2

While travelling home on the bus you come across a note that has been left on the seat. On the note is a table with some codes that correspond to different words. You then spot some codes that have been drawn on the seat in front. You decide to use the translations of the codes on the note to solve the puzzle.

C	Increase	122	Transport	555	Ticket
D	Plural	158	Person	643	Money
F	Generalise	171	Car	787	Sad
J	Forward	219	Purchase	788	Face
N	Past	266	Sun	865	Large
R	Personalise	302	Cloud	897	Holiday
T	Opposite	402	Two	988	Body

Question 1: In the future driving will be more expensive.

    A.   CN, C 643, 171 555

    B.   F (171 122), C 643, TN

    C.   CJ, C 643, R F(171 122)

    D.   TN, 122 (R 171), C 643

    E.   F, 171 122, C 643

Question 2: Booking my holiday made me smile.

    A.   219 555 897, (T 787)

    B.   219 R (897 122), (T 787) 788

    C.   R ((122 897), T 787)

    D.   219 R (555, 897), R (T 787) 788

Question 3: The king is very rich and has bought two cars.

    A.   C 158, C (C 643), 219 (402 171)

    B.   F 158, C D 643, 219 (402 171)

    C.   C 158, F 643, 219, 402 171

    D.   402 (C 158, C 643, 219 171)

    E.   C 158, D 643, D 171, 219

Example Set 2: Answers and Explanations

Question 1: B. F (171 122), C 643, TN

    A.   CN is incorrect as this would code for 'increase past' not 'future'. The combination C 643 must be correct as it is present in all answer options and codes for 'increase money'. The use of 'ticket' makes no sense and the wrong code has been used.

    B.   This is the correct answer. But remember the order of the codes doesn't matter as long as brackets are preserved and grouped codes remain grouped together.

    C.   'Increase forward' could code for future and would work, as would 'increase money'. However, there is the introduction of 'R – personalise' which isn't in the sentence. This would incorrectly relate the car/driving to me.

    D.   Again this code incorrectly introduces 'R – personalise', making it 'in the future driving *my* car'.

    E.   There is no representation of tense in this answer, thereby making it incomplete.

Question 2: D. 219 R (555, 897), R (T 787) 788

A. There is no representation of 'personalise' in the first part of the sentence, so this code does not translate into 'my holiday'. The last part of the code – '(T 787)' – is not a good translation for smile as it would translate as 'opposite sad', which would be happy.

B. The first part would conceivably be correct, although not the best translation. However, there is no representation of 'personalise' in relation to 'smile'.

C. Although the 'personalise' relates to the entire sentence there is no representation of 'booking'. The last part is not a good translation for 'smile', as it would translate as 'opposite sad' which would be happy.

D. Correct

Question 3: A. C 158, C (C 643), 219 (402 171)

A. Correct

B. The start of the code, 'F 158', would translate as 'generalise person'. If you generalise something you make it less specific, not more specific, and as such this would not translate to 'king'.

C. Generalising money would not accurately translate as 'very rich', as there is nothing to denote 'very'.

D. The brackets and codes are in the wrong place. In this code 'two' would be multiplied into each component in the bracket, generating 'two kings'. This would be incorrect. Again, there is no notion of 'very rich' as 'increase money' could certainly mean 'rich' but not 'very rich'.

E. In this option there is no mention of 'very' rich. There is a plural of 'two', relating to 'car', making it incorrect.

Add New Words

The final question style comprises only one or two out of the 28 DA questions that you will be presented with. You are presented with a sentence followed by five words. You need to select which **two** out of the five words you would want to add to your existing table of codes, in order to make it possible to code for the given sentence.

Strategy for Add New Words

1. Cross reference the five words with your existing table of codes

   Although you will not have any of the five words in your table of codes you might have a very similar word or a synonym which you could use in its place, thereby making it unnecessary to add that word.

2. Create words using powerful operators

   There may be words in the sentence which, although they aren't in your table of codes, you can generate by combining existing codes with powerful operators. For instance, if you needed the word 'king' but had 'increase' and 'man' in your table, you could conceivably create 'king' by using 'increase man'.

3. Add one of the words

After trying Steps 1 and 2, if you still have more than two words left to choose from you must ask yourself: 'Does combining one of the remaining words with an existing code or powerful operator achieve the desired result?' When adopting this technique, it is vital that you always look for the simplest and neatest fit, requiring the fewest number of steps and assumptions.

Example Set 3

We will use the same table of codes as used in Example Set 2.

C	Increase	122	Transport	555	Ticket
D	Plural	158	Person	643	Money
F	Generalise	171	Car	787	Sad
J	Forward	219	Purchase	788	Face
N	Negative	266	Sun	865	Large
R	Personalise	302	Cloud	897	Holiday
T	Opposite	402	Two	988	Body

Question 1: Which **two** words have to be added to the code to create the following phrase?

Thunderstorms delayed the flight by hours as the wings were damaged.

    A.   Thunderstorm

    B.   Delayed

    C.   Flight

    D.   Hours

    E.   Wing

Question 2: Which **two** words have to be added to the code to create the following phrase?

Monkeys are happy when they are given lots of fruit and bananas.

    A.   Monkey

    B.   Happy

    C.   Give

    D.   Fruit

    E.   Banana

Example Set 3: Answers and Explanations

Question 1: D and E (hours and wing)

A. You could create 'thunderstorm' using numerous combinations, such as 'increase negative cloud' or 'plural increase cloud'.

B. 'Delayed' is in itself not possible to create. However, if you were to add 'hours' to your code then you could easily create 'delayed' using 'increase hours'.

C. 'Flight' could be created using 'generalise cloud transport', among other alternatives.

D. Not possible to create.

E. Not possible to create.

Question 2: A and E (monkey and banana)

A. Not possible to create.

B. You have the codes for 'opposite' and 'sad' so by combining these together you could create 'happy'.

C. You have the codes for 'opposite' and 'purchase' so you could combine them to create 'give'.

D. 'Fruit' is not possible to create using your table of codes. However, if you add 'banana' and combine it with 'generalise' you could easily create 'fruit'.

E. Not possible to create. (You could add 'fruit' and use this to 'opposite generalise fruit' and make 'banana'. But this is not a neat fit compared to other available options.)

Time for some practice! Try answering the following **28 Practice Questions** containing a mixture of the three question styles. You have 31 minutes to answer all questions. Detailed explanations are provided. Good luck!

Practice Sets

Question Set 1

While walking through a forest on holiday in Scandinavia you discover an old, previously undisturbed runestone beneath some bushes. As you gently brush away the dirt you see there is a series of codes consisting of letters and numbers running along the edges of the stone. On the back of the stone you discover a table where different codes correlate to words. You set about trying to decode the cryptic messages.

A	Plural	008	Take	502	Living
B	Generalise	152	Fire	676	Silver
C	Opposite	177	Riding	682	Man
E	Personalise	190	Viking	722	Church
H	Negative	200	Wedding	746	Singing
L	Increase	269	House	808	Two
M		311	Gold	818	Person
O		324	Horse	820	Shout

Example 1: (C L) 190, (L 746) 722

    A.   The happy Viking sang loudly in the church.

    B.   The happy Viking sang in the large church.

    C.   The happy Viking was singing loudly in the large church.

    D.   More Vikings were singing loudly in the churches.

    E.   Singing loudly in the church made the Viking happy.

Although all the codes above link to the answer it's important to look at the brackets – the opposite and negative are linked (which in this context must code for 'happy'). Furthermore, the increase is linked to sing and not church so 'large church' or 'churches' must be wrong. The correct answer is therefore A.

Example 2: L 682, 502, (C L) 269

    A.   The men lived in small houses.

    B.   Many men lived in a few small houses.

    C.   The tall man lived in a small house.

    D.   The tall men are living in small houses.

    E.   The men were living in their houses.

In this code 'increase man' could either mean 'tall man' or 'men' but as you only have one code for increase it could not mean both. Similarly 'opposite increase' could mean small or fewer, but not both, so when combining these points only answer C could be correct.

Question 1: (L 269) 152, H 502 (E 324)

    A. The large fire in the house killed my horse.

    B. A large fire burned down my house killing the horses.

    C. The house fire killed my horse.

    D. A fire in the mansion killed my horse.

    E. The large fire in the palace killed my horse.

Question 2: A (B 190), 008 (B (311, 676)), 722

    A. The Vikings stole gold and silver from churches.

    B. The Vikings stole the treasure from the church.

    C. The Vikings took treasure from the churches.

    D. The warriors took the gold and silver from the church.

    E. The warriors took the treasure from the church.

Question 3: 746 (A 818), L 722, 746, E 200

    A. The choir sang in the Cathedral for my wedding.

    B. The choir sang many songs in the church for my wedding.

    C. The choir sang loudly in the church for my wedding.

    D. Everyone was singing in the Cathedral for my wedding.

    E. The group were singing in the big church for my wedding.

Question 4: L (808 818), C 008, B (818, 311)

    A. People should spread their wealth in society.

    B. More than two people have taken the people's gold.

    C. The Royal couple gave the people gold.

    D. Wealthy people have given money to other people.

    E. Everyone can take gold from the people.

Question 5: (C 682) 820, 808 682, 177 (A 324)

    A. The woman shouted at the two men riding their horse.

    B. The woman shouted at the two men riding horses.

    C. The boy was shouted at by the two men riding horses.

    D. The boy shouted at the two men on their horses.

    E. Two men shouted at a woman riding a horse.

Question 6: E (808 818), 502, L 269

    A. Two people live in my large house.

    B. Several couples live in the house.

C. We all live in my large house.

D. Two of us live in a large house.

E. The couple lives in a large house.

Question 7: A 190, 152, A 269, 008, B (311, 676)

A. The Vikings set fire to the village and took the valuables.

B. The Vikings set many houses on fire taking the gold and silver.

C. The Vikings set many fires burning down the houses and taking the treasure.

D. The Vikings set fire to the village after stealing the gold and silver.

E. The Vikings set fire to and burned down the village taking all the valuables.

Question 8: L 682, E (C 008), 676, E 200

A. People gave silver at my wedding.

B. Several men took my silver at my wedding.

C. The tall man gave me money at the wedding.

D. Many people have given me money at weddings.

E. The old man gave me silver for my wedding.

Question 9: H 682, 008, E (808 324), 269

A. The thief stole the two horses from the house.

B. The man is angry as someone took his horses from his house.

C. The depressed man took the two horses to the house.

D. The sad man took his two horses to the house.

E. The thief stole the two horses from my house.

Question 10: The king rode his horse to the palace.

A. L 682, 177, E (324, (L 269))

B. L 682, 177 E 324, E (L 269)

C. L 682, 177, E 324, L 269

D. B 190, 177, 324, E 269

Question 11: My father lives in a bungalow.

A. E (L 682), 502, H 269

B. E (L 682), 502, C (L 269)

C. B 818, 502, L (H 269)

D. L 682, 502, C (L 269)

E. L 682, 502, L (H 269)

Question 12: The two Vikings rode their big horses to the stable.

    A. 808 (190 177), L (A 324), E (269 324)

    B. 808 (190 177), E, L (A 324), E (269 324)

    C. (808 190) 177, E 324 A, (269 324)

    D. (808 190) 177, E 324, L(269 324)

    E. (808 190) 177, E (L 324 A), 269 324

Question 13: The man stole the woman's engagement ring.

    A. H 682, 008, C 682, B (311 676)

    B. 682, H 008, (C 682), E (200 676)

    C. 682, H 008, E (C 682), B (200 676)

    D. H (682 008), C 682, B (E (311 676))

Question 14: Which **two** words have to be added to the code to create the following phrase?

The woman was angry at her husband for crashing their car into a river.

    A. Angry

    B. Husband

    C. Crashing

    D. Car

    E. River

As you continue to explore you find a second runestone nearby which contains even more codes. When combining the two codes you now have the following table:

A	Plural	008	Take	502	Living
B	Generalise	152	Fire	676	Silver
C	Opposite	177	Riding	682	Man
E	Personalise	190	Viking	722	Church
H	Negative	200	Wedding	746	Singing
L	Increase	269	House	808	Two
M	Command	311	Gold	818	Person
O	Emotion	324	Horse	820	Shout
R	Future	347	Book	845	Enter
T	Positive	399	Carriage	898	Translate
U	Pay	444	Pub	923	Nearby
X	Crop	456	Field	967	Taxation
Z	Destroy	499	Servant	971	Road

Question 15: (R (L 682)), L 967, A 818

    A. The next king will raise the taxes for the people.

    B. In the future the king will raise taxes.

    C. The king will raise taxes for the people.

    D. In the future, taxes will rise as there will be more people.

    E. The future king will raise taxes.

Question 16: 967 818, M, (C 682) U, E (808 499)

    A. The woman ordered her two servants to pay tax.

    B. The woman was ordered to pay her two servants tax.

    C. The tax man ordered the woman's two servants to pay tax.

    D. The tax man ordered the woman to pay her two servants.

    E. The tax man made the two servant boys pay their tax.

Question 17: The crops failed in both the big fields.

    A. X, H 502, 808 456

    B. X A, C 502, A L 456

    C. A X, B O, 808 (L 456)

    D. X A, H 502, 808 456 A

    E. A X, C 502, 808 (L 456)

Question 18: (T O) (C 682), E 177 324, 722

    A. The happy woman rode to church.

    B. The cheerful woman enjoys riding her horse to church.

    C. The woman is happy riding her horses to church.

    D. The happy boy rode his horse to the church.

    E. The small man rode the cheerful horse to church.

Question 19: The man paid the two servants to translate books.

    A. 682 U, A 499, 898 (808 347)

    B. 682 U, 808 499, 898 (A 347)

    C. 682, U (808 499), 898 347

    D. 682, U 499, 898 (808 347)

Question 20: A 499, 177 E (A 234), 456, 808 456

    A. The servant rode his horse across the field.

    B. The servants rode across the two fields.

    C. The servants rode their horses across the two fields.

D. The servants rode their two horses across the fields.

E. The servants rode horses across both fields.

Question 21: 190, 845 444, (H O) 820 (444 682)

A. The Viking entered the pub and angrily shouted at the barman.

B. The Viking entered the depressing pub and shouted at the customers.

C. The angry Viking entered the pub shouting at the customers.

D. The Viking entered the pub quietly talking to the barman.

E. The Vikings quietly spoke to the customers in the pub.

Question 22: People with a lot of wealth pay higher taxes.

A. A 818, L ((311 676) (L 967))

B. A 818, L (311 676), U 967

C. A 818, L B (311 676), U (L 967)

D. A 818, A 311, U (L 967)

Question 23: L 152 Z, E L 269, H 502 (A E 324)

A. A large fire destroyed the large house and killed my horses.

B. The large fire destroyed my mansion and killed my horses.

C. Several fires destroyed my houses and killed my horse.

D. Large fires destroyed my house and killed my horses.

E. The fires destroyed my mansions and killed my horses.

Question 24: ((L 190) M), E (A 682), 177, E (A 324)

A. The Vikings were ordered by the people to ride their horses.

B. The Vikings commanded the people to ride their horses.

C. The chieftain instructed his men to ride their horses.

D. The warlord ordered his men to leave on their horses.

E. Vikings are strong people who ride horses.

Question 25: The crops thrived in the fields near the two churches.

A. A X, 502, A 456, 923, (808 722)

B. A X, (T 502), 456, 808 722

C. A X, (L 502), 923, A (456, 722)

D. (A X), L 502, 923 456, (808 722)

E. (A X) (L 502), A 456, 923, 808 722

Question 26: A (L (C 682)), C 820, 808 682, 923 444

A. The women quietly spoke to the two men near the pub.

B. The fat women shouted at the two men outside the pub.

C. The fat woman spoke to the men near the pub.

D. The tall women spoke to the two men near the pub.

E. The very tall women were talking to the two men near the pub.

Question 27: L 682, 200, (T O) (200 (C 682)), (C L) 722

A. The tall man was happy as he married his fiancé in a small church.

B. The tall man married the happy bride in the small church.

C. Some men are happy to get married in a small church but others are not.

D. The men married the happy brides in a small church.

E. The fat man married the happy bride in the beautiful church.

Question 28: Which **two** words have to be added to the code to create the following phrase?

The old man polished his expensive silver knives and cutlery set.

A. Old

B. Polished

C. Expensive

D. Knives

E. Cutlery

Answers

Question 1: D. A fire in the mansion killed my horse.

The literal translation of the code is: (increase house) fire, negative living (personalise horse)

A.   'L 269 – increase house' is contained within brackets and so must remain linked to each other. The 'large' therefore refers to the house and not the fire.

B.   Once again the 'large' must refer to the house and not the fire and in the code horse is singular, while in this answer it is plural.

C.   There is no representation of 'L – increase', making it an incomplete answer.

D.   Correct

E.   Increase has been used twice in this answer – once to make palace (increase house) and once to describe the fire, yet increase is only represented once in the code.

Question 2: E. The warriors took the treasure from the church.

The literal translation of the code is: plural (generalise Viking), take (generalise (gold, silver)), church

A.   The start of the code has incorrectly missed out 'generalise'. If you generalise something you make it less specific, and therefore answers containing 'Viking' cannot be correct. This option has also not generalised gold and silver and has a plural for churches, which should be singular.

B.   The start of the code has incorrectly missed out 'generalise'. If you generalise something you make it less specific and therefore answers containing 'Viking' cannot be correct. The rest of the translation is correct.

C.   The start of the code has incorrectly missed out 'generalise'. If you generalise something you make it less specific and therefore answers containing 'Viking' cannot be correct. Church is singular in the code but plural in this answer and so this option cannot be correct.

D.   Generalising Viking could create warrior, however, this option forgets to generalise gold and silver and so cannot be correct.

E.   Correct

Question 3: A. The choir sang in the Cathedral for my wedding.

The literal translation of the code is: singing (plural person), increase church, singing, personalise wedding

A.   Correct (as this takes into account that singing is represented twice in the code – once creating choir and once as sang).

B.   There is no representation in the code for 'songs' and increase refers to church anyway so to say 'many songs' is incorrect for two reasons.

C.   The increase refers to church and not singing therefore 'sang loudly' is incorrect.

D.   This answer has only used '746 – singing' once. In the previous answers the first singing has been used to create 'choir'; however, this answer simply uses 'everyone' and is therefore incomplete, having only used singing once.

E.   This answer has only used '746 – singing' once. In the previous answers the first singing has been used to create 'choir'; however, this answer simply uses 'the group' and is therefore incomplete, having only used singing once.

Question 4: C. The Royal couple gave the people gold.

The literal translation of the code is: increase (two person), opposite take, generalise person, gold

A.   Although 'people' isn't a good translation of 'increase (two person)' there are other errors in this answer, such as the extra word 'should' and 'wealth in society'. The 'generalise' refers to person and not gold and, as such, although society could be created by 'generalise person', wealth is a leap from gold. Overall, this answer contains many smaller ambiguous errors and therefore is not an ideal fit.

B.   The code codes for 'opposite take', whereas this answer has not used opposite and therefore kept 'take' instead of creating 'give'.

C.   Correct (two person is a couple and increase is used to increase greatness/stature to make Royal).

D.   There is no code for wealth relating to people in the opening part of this so there is an extra word. Although not ideal, 'gold' could be used as money but this would be ambiguous.

E.   This answer is missing a representation for 'C – opposite' and is therefore incomplete.

Question 5: B. The woman shouted at the two men riding horses.

The literal translation of the code is: (opposite man) shout, two man, riding (plural horse)

A.   This option has introduced 'their' into the answer but there is no personalise in the code. Furthermore horse should be plural and not singular.

B.   Correct

C.   Shout is grouped with 'opposite man' so although 'boy' is an acceptable translation of 'opposite man' it should be the boy shouted at, not the other way round.

D.   This option has introduced 'their' into the answer but there is no personalise in the code.

E.   Shout is grouped with 'opposite man' so it should be the woman who shouted at the two men, not the other way round and horse should be plural and not singular.

Question 6: D. Two of us live in a large house.

The literal translation of the code is: personalise (two person), living, increase house

A.   The code for personalise refers to two people and not house so 'my large house' is incorrect.

B.   The increase is grouped with house, not at the start of the sentence, so it should be large house not increase (as in number) of couples. There is also no representation of 'personalise'.

C.   'Personalise (two person)' does not translate well to 'we' and this answer also uses 'personalise' twice as it appears a second time as 'my large house'.

D.   Correct

E.   There is no representation of 'personalise' in this answer.

Question 7: A. The Vikings set fire to the village and took the valuables.

The literal translation of the code is: plural Viking, fire, plural house, take, generalise (gold, silver)

    A. Correct

    B. This option has not generalised 'gold and silver' at the end and is therefore incomplete.

    C. Although most parts of this translation are correct 'plural' has been used once too many a time. There is a code for plural relating to Viking and house but not to fire (which is singular). The answer has also used 'fire' twice – once in fires and once in burning.

    D. This option has not generalised 'gold and silver' at the end and is therefore incomplete.

    E. This answer has also used 'fire' twice – once in 'set fire' and once in 'burned'.

Question 8: E. The old man gave me silver for my wedding.

The literal translation of the code is: increase man, personalise (opposite take), silver, personalise wedding

    A. Although 'increase man' might mean people this would be a poor translation of the code given there is a code for person. There is, however, no representation of personalise in the context of 'give' (remember personalise appears twice in the code).

    B. This option has not used 'opposite take' to create give but instead kept the code as 'take'.

    C. Silver could be interpreted as money; however, this answer doesn't utilise the second personalise in relation to wedding.

    D. Many people would be a poor and inaccurate translation of 'increase man'. This answer also doesn't use the second 'personalise' and weddings should be singular and not plural.

    E. Correct

Question 9: D. The sad man took his two horses to the house.

The literal translation of the code is: negative man, take, personalise (two horse), house

    A. A negative man could be a thief but this answer is incomplete because there is no representation of 'personalise' anywhere in the answer.

    B. There is an extra word 'someone' in the answer, which is not represented in the code.

    C. There is no representation of 'personalise' in this answer.

    D. Correct

    E. The 'personalise' has been combined with house instead of 'two horses'. Remember that brackets must be multiplied out correctly and items within brackets remain linked.

Question 10: C. L 682, 177, E 324, L 269

    A. The brackets are wrong in the final part of the sentence. The 'personalise' therefore refers to both horse and 'increase house', thereby making it 'his horse to *his* palace', while the question states *the* palace.

B. There is an extra 'E – personalise' in this code, making the final part 'his palace' not 'the palace'.

C. Correct

D. There are numerous errors in this code. The 'generalise Viking' does not code for king, the 'personalise' refers to house and not horse and there is no code changing house to palace.

Question 11: B. E (L 682), 502, C (L 269)

A. The first part of the sentence is correct but 'H 269 – negative house' doesn't necessarily code for a bungalow and this would be the second best answer.

B. Correct

C. 'Generalise person' would not code for 'father' and there is no representation of the code 'personalise'. The last part of the sentence, 'increase negative house', doesn't make much sense.

D. There is no representation of 'my' in the opening part of this code.

E. There is no representation of 'my' in the opening part of this code and the last part of the sentence, 'increase negative house', doesn't make much sense.

Question 12: E. (808 190) 177, E (L 324 A), 269 324

A. The first part of the code works; however, there is no representation of 'their' horse, instead the 'personalise' is incorrectly referring to the stable and not the horse.

B. This answer option has a 'personalise' too many and, although it could create 'their horses', it would also incorrectly create 'their stable'.

C. There is no representation of 'big' in the context of the horse and the horse is singular and not plural.

D. The 'increase' is incorrectly coupled with stable, creating 'large stable' not large horses.

E. Correct

Question 13: B. 682, H 008, (C 682), E (200 676)

A. In this code the negative refers to man not take, so would technically code for 'the thief took' not 'the man stole'. Generalising gold and silver doesn't create engagement ring and there is also no element of personalisation of this object.

B. Correct

C. The first two groups make sense; however, in the second group, the 'personalise' is referring to the woman and not the ring. Although this answer is not catastrophically wrong, it equally is not the best fit answer.

D. The main problem in this code is in the last section 'B (E (311 676)) – generalise (personalise (gold silver))', which does not have any representation of wedding or engagement.

Question 14: D and E (car and river)

A. Angry could be represented as 'personalise fire'.

B. Husband could be represented as 'wedding man'.

C. Crashing is possible to create if you add car to the list. By combining negative (car riding) for instance this could mean crash.

D. Not possible

E. Not possible

Question 15: A. The next king will raise the taxes for the people.

The literal translation of the code is: (future (increase man)), increase taxation, plural person

A. Correct

B. The future is referring to 'increase man' and not the whole sentence. Therefore, it must be 'the next king' or 'the future king', not generally in the futures. There is also no representation of 'plural person' in this answer.

C. The future has incorrectly been linked to the whole sentence, which is an example of incorrectly multiplying out the brackets. The future refers to 'increase man', as is contained within brackets, so must translate as 'the next or future king'.

D. The future once again incorrectly refers to the whole sentence and there is no representation of 'increase man'.

E. There is no representation of the last part of the sentence, 'plural person', so this answer is incomplete.

Question 16: D. The tax man ordered the woman to pay her two servants.

The literal translation of the code is: taxation person, command, (opposite man) pay, personalise (two servants)

A. The 'pay' is linked to the woman and not the servants in the code. There is also no translation of '967 818 – taxation person'.

B. Again there is no translation of '967 818 – taxation person'.

C. The word tax has featured twice in this answer but only once in the code and the 'pay' is linked to the woman and not the servants.

D. Correct

E. The word 'tax' is featured twice in this answer but only once in the code and, although 'opposite man' could translate as 'boy', this has been incorrectly linked with servant.

Question 17: E. A X, C 502, 808 (L 456)

A. There is no concept of plural in relation to crop nor of size in relation to the field.

B. Although almost correct there is no representation of 'both', i.e. two in this answer; instead, simply 'plural', which is less specific.

C. 'Generalise emotion' does not translate to 'failed'. The extra code 'A – plural' at the end is unnecessary as the code 'two' is already present in relation to the fields.

D. This is similar to answer A and, although the crops is now plural, there is no representation of 'big' in relation to fields in this answer.

E. Correct

Question 18: D. The happy boy rode his horse to the church.

The literal translation of the code is: (positive emotion) (opposite man), personalise riding horse, church

    A.   There is no representation of 'E – personalise' in this answer, making it incomplete.

    B.   This answer has used both 'cheerful' and 'enjoys', thereby using the code 'positive emotion' twice instead of once.

    C.   This answer is almost a good fit; however, horses is singular in the code yet plural in this option.

    D.   Correct

    E.   The 'positive emotion' has incorrectly been linked to horse and not 'the small man' and there is no representation of personalise anywhere in the answer.

Question 19: B. 682 U, 808 499, 898 (A 347)

    A.   The 'two' and 'plural' are in the wrong places in this code incorrectly making 'the servants' and 'two books'.

    B.   Correct

    C.   There is no representation of plural in relation to book here, making it singular in answer option.

    D.   The servant in this answer option is singular and instead the 'two' is referring to books.

Question 20: C. The servants rode their horses across the two fields.

The literal translation of the code is: plural servant, riding personalised (plural horse), two field

    A.   Servant is singular but should be plural and there is no representation of 'two' in relation to fields.

    B.   Part of the code 'A 234 – plural horse' is missing from this answer.

    C.   Correct

    D.   In this option the position of plural (in relation to the horse) and two have been swapped round incorrectly giving 'two horses' and 'fields'.

    E.   There is no representation of 'personalise' in this response, making it incomplete.

Question 21: A. The Viking entered the pub and angrily shouted at the barman.

The literal translation of the code is: Viking, enter pub, (negative emotion) shout (pub man)

    A.   Correct

    B.   The 'negative emotion' is linked with shout and not pub so it is incorrect to say 'depressing pub'.

    C.   Although the first part of the sentence could work the last part refers to 'customers' as a plural, yet there is no code for making it plural.

    D.   The 'negative' refers to emotion and not 'shout', so it can't downgrade the shout to talk.

E. The 'negative' refers to emotion and not 'shout', so it can't downgrade the shout to talk and there is an incorrect plural in relation to customer (which is a poor translation of 'bar man').

Question 22: C. A 818, L B (311 676), U (L 967)

A. This code would translate as 'people increase wealth increase tax' but there is no notion of 'pay' in the answer.

B. This answer is missing 'higher' in relation to taxes as the last part simply decodes as 'pay taxation'.

C. Correct

D. Although the last part of the translation would work, the middle part would simply decode as 'plural gold'. This might be taken to mean 'lot of wealth'; however, it is not as good or accurate a translation as option C.

Question 23: B. The large fire destroyed my mansion and killed my horses.

The literal translation of the code is: increase fire destroy, personalise increase house, negative living (plural personalise horse).

A. This option has not used the first 'personalise', which relates to the house.

B. Correct

C. Although the first part of the sentence would work (using increase to increase the number of both fire and house) there is an error in the last part as horse is singular but should be plural.

D. Large fires is not possible – either increase refers to the size of the fire or the number but can't be both. There is no representation of 'increase' in relation to the house.

E. It is not possible to create 'mansions' as either the increase can be used to create mansion or houses (plural) but not both – this would have used increase twice.

Question 24: C. The chieftain instructed his men to ride their horses.

The literal translation of the code is: ((increase Viking) command), personalise (plural man), riding, personalise (plural horse).

A. 'Vikings' and 'command' are both within brackets and so must therefore remain linked together. In this answer option the 'command' has been linked with the next part of the sentence.

B. This option has only used 'personalise' once and there is therefore no representation of 'personalise' in relation to 'the people'.

C. Correct

D. Although 'increase Viking' might translate to 'warlord', 'riding' doesn't neatly translate as 'leave'. This translation would work but has two poor translations of the code and is therefore not the best answer.

E. 'Command' has been incorrectly translated as 'strong' and there is no representation of their either in relation to people or to horses.

Question 25: E. (A X) (L 502), A 456, 923, 808 722

A. This answer is good; however, there is nothing to suggest 'thrive' as opposed to simply 'living'. The code 'living' would need to be combined with another code such as 'increase' or 'positive' to create 'thrive'.

B. 'T 502 – positive living' could certainly be interpreted as 'thrive'; however, there is nothing in this answer to make field plural.

C. This answer is incorrect as 'plural' has been grouped with both field (correct) and church (incorrect – should be two, not plural).

D. Once again there is no 'plural' in relation to field, thereby making this option incorrect.

E. Correct

Question 26: D. The tall women spoke to the two men near the pub.

The literal translation of the code is: plural (increase (opposite man)), opposite shout, two man, nearby pub

A. The first part of the code is for 'plural (increase (opposite man))'; however, this answer option has no representation of 'increase' and has simply left it as 'women'. 'Opposite shout' could mean talk; however, there is an extra adjective here – quietly.

B. This sentence is incorrect as it has not used the code 'opposite' in relation to shout.

C. There are two main errors in this answer. First, there is no representation of 'plural' in relation to 'fat woman' and second there is no representation of 'two' in relation to the men.

D. Correct

E. There is an extra adjective in the opening part of this sentence 'very', which is not coded for as it would require an extra 'increase'.

Question 27: B. The tall man married the happy bride in the small church.

The literal translation of the code is: increase man, wedding, (positive emotion) (wedding (opposite man)), (opposite increase) church

A. The 'positive emotion' is linked with the bride/fiancé and not with the tall man so this option is incorrect.

B. Correct

C. This sentence doesn't take into account the brackets and that '(wedding (opposite man))' would in this case code for bride or fiancé.

D. In this option 'bride' has become plural yet is singular in the code, thereby making it incorrect.

E. The first part of this option is correct; however, 'opposite increase' would not code for 'beautiful'.

Question 28: B and D (polished and knives)

A. The 'old man' could be represented simply as 'increase man' with increase referring to age.

B. Not possible

C. Expensive could be created in different ways, such as 'increase pay' or 'generalise increase gold' etc.

D. Not possible

E. Initially this is not possible to code; however, if you were to add 'knives' to your table of codes then you could generate cutlery using 'generalise knives'.

CHAPTER 5

Situational Judgement Test

Overview

The Situational Judgement Test (SJT) is the newest component to be added to the UKCAT exam, having been introduced in 2013. It presents students with a range of hypothetical life and work-related scenarios to assess how they deal with them. The scenarios focus on:

- Ethical and moral dilemmas
- Managing difficult emotional situations
- Conflict resolution
- Integrity
- Honesty
- Team working skills

Situational judgement testing is becoming increasingly popular in the world of medicine. You will be tested again using SJTs at medical school, as part of your FY1 application and for entry into certain postgraduate speciality training programmes.

In 2014 there was an error in the marking of the SJT section of the exam, forcing the UKCAT board to withdraw this section from the exam, and universities were instructed not to take the SJT score into account. Situational judgement testing will however feature once again in 2015.

Format of the Section

This section consists of 67 questions split across 20 scenarios. Each scenario has between three and six associated questions. You have a generous 27 minutes (including 1 minute of reading time) to complete the section. This leaves you with approximately 23 seconds per question. Although this doesn't sound like much, students often feel that this section is the least time pressured in the UKCAT.

There are two types of tasks:

- Rating the appropriateness of a response to the scenario
- Rating how important it is to undertake an action in the context of a scenario

Scoring

The scoring used in the situational judgement section is completely different to the other four sections of the UKCAT. In other sections, the correct answer scores one mark. In SJT, the best answer scores the most points, but subsequent answers may also score points. You will therefore accumulate points through the section, picking up more points the more consistently you get the best – or close to the best – answer. Your raw score is then converted into a 'band', ranging from Band 1 (highest) to Band 4 (lowest). This is then presented as a standalone score. It is *not* combined with your score from the other four sections.

What does this mean? Each university will look at the SJT score independently from your scores for the other four sections. Many universities do not look at the SJT score. For those that do, a Band 1 or 2 score should be sufficient to meet their criteria.

Top Tip: Always use your UKCAT score strategically. If your SJT score is lower than you hoped for, look at applying to universities who do not consider the SJT score.

General Strategy

In order to be successful in SJT you must remember some golden rules that apply to both question types:

1. They are assessing your actions, not the scenario. The scenarios are designed to be challenging and may involve you having acted irresponsibly. The aim of SJT is to assess how you *respond*. You could have done something awful in the scenario but the way in which you deal with it can still be excellent.

2. Never make assumptions. In SJT, it is tempting to keep asking what if. As a result, you might assume things that are not stated or implied. Do not assume anything to be the case unless it is written. Base your response purely on the facts you have.

3. You do not need any pre-existing medical knowledge. The UKCAT is meant to assess aptitude, rather than knowledge. SJT is no exception. Although a basic understanding of how to deal with difficult situations and ethics will help you, you will not be expected to have any specific medical knowledge.

4. Always ask yourself: 'What does the examiner want me to do?' Often, what we should do and what we actually do are completely different. Our judgement may become clouded, as a scenario may be based around a friend rather than a stranger.

However, it is important to stay impartial and consider the 'textbook' approach to tackling any scenario.

5. For each scenario you can use each answer option as many or as few times as you wish.

6. Each question within a scenario is completely independent from all other questions. Answers are not dependent on how you responded to previous questions.

7. The actions provided are not 'complete'. Sometimes students are put off from selecting strong answers (such as 'very appropriate' or 'very inappropriate') as the action described on its own does not seem strong enough. However, you should never judge the response as if it is the only action taken.

Appropriateness Questions

Appropriateness questions ask you to rate how appropriate you think a response is, in the context of the scenario. You have four options to choose from:

- A very appropriate thing to do
- Appropriate, but not ideal
- Inappropriate, but not awful
- A very inappropriate thing to do

Strategy for Appropriateness Questions

Always read the scenario first. In SJT, unlike other sections of the UKCAT, it is impossible to answer the questions without having read the scenario beforehand. Fortunately, the scenarios tend to be quite short and don't take long to read.

Students often find it hard to choose between the various options. Getting to grips with how to differentiate between the answers can seem tricky. When you analyse the answers, you might frequently find that some are positive, some are negative, and some contain a mixture of positive and negative elements:

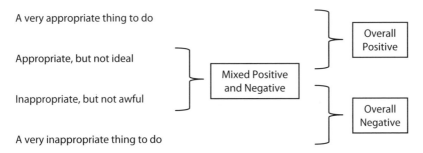

To help you decide on the correct answer it is best to adopt an algorithm. First, you must decide if you think the action is positive or negative overall. The second step is to decide if the action is 'pure' or 'mixed', i.e. are all components of the action positive or negative? Or is there a mixture of positive and negative elements?

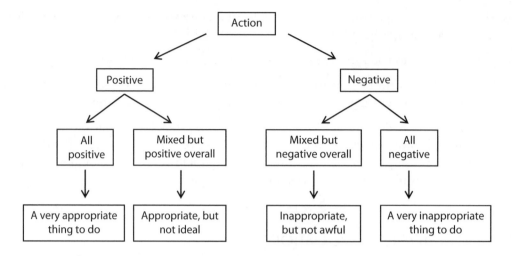

If you stick to this principle you will find it much easier to approach appropriateness questions. The real challenge arises when you have a mixture of positive and negative and you need to decide which one is stronger.

> **Top Tip:** Some students (and books) recommend always choosing the mixed options instead of the 'very' options, as even if you are wrong you are likely to be close to the correct answer and therefore pick up some points. This does not work!

Importance Questions

Importance questions ask you to rate how important you think a response is, in the context of the scenario. You have four options to choose from:

- Very important
- Important
- Of minor importance
- Not important at all

It is crucial that you understand the definitions of the terms correctly in order to identify the correct response. Following are some modified definitions of the terms:

Very important: You *must* take this into account.

Important: You *should* take this into account.

Of minor importance: You *may* take this into account.

Not important at all: You should *not* take this into account.

Items that are crucial to undertake or consider are therefore 'very important'. Items that are important to consider, although not essential, are 'important'. If the item is something that you can take into account but equally it is completely acceptable even if you do not, then it is 'of minor importance'. If the item is negative, and one that should not be enacted, or even taken into account, then it is 'not important at all'.

We will now look at some theory and questions designed to help you decide between the various answer options.

Example Scenario 1

You are a first-year medical student at university, and to help fund your tuition fees, you work part time at a local restaurant. You soon begin to notice that some items, including money from the tip jar, have started to disappear and you suspect that one of your co-workers is stealing them.

How appropriate is the following response?

You decide to confront the person you think is responsible, threatening to report them to the management unless they return the items.

A. A very appropriate thing to do

B. Appropriate, but not ideal

C. Inappropriate, but not awful

D. A very inappropriate thing to do

Example Scenario 1: Answer and Explanation

In this case, the correct answer is 'Inappropriate, but not awful'. It is obvious that you have good intentions, both for yourself and fellow staff, to stop the stealing. You are also giving the person a chance to come clean and return the items. However, remember you only *suspect* they are responsible. As such, you could be offering an ultimatum (return the items or I report you) to someone who is innocent. There is clearly a mixture of positive and negative here.

Another major factor in helping you decide on the correct answer is the tone of your response. You 'confront' and 'threaten' the person in question. Confrontational and threatening behaviour is clearly not what the medical schools are looking for. It will be difficult to justify an overall positive response for actions that utilise these words.

Choice of Vocabulary

It is vital that you pay close attention to the wording used to describe the action. This will help guide you as to whether or not the response is positive or negative. Following is a table of positive and negative words:

Positive		Negative	
Truthful	Propose	Threaten	Abuse
Honest	Encourage	Shout	Refuse
Open	Explore	Intimidate	Hide
Calm	Listen	Avoid	Blame
Support	Suggest	Confront	Shun
Recommend	Boost	Impatient	Accuse

If your action contains mainly positive words, then it is likely the action will be positive overall. Actions that contain negative words are unlikely to be positive overall. Changing the choice of wording has a drastic impact on the answer choice. Consider the above scenario again. But this time ask yourself how appropriate the following response is:

You sit down with the person in question, calmly voicing your concerns to him, and explore his side of the story.

In contrast, using words such as 'calmly' and 'exploring' gives a very positive tone to your response, making it very appropriate overall.

Example Scenario 2

You are sitting in your sixth form common room when a friend approaches you, upset. He has been having trouble with his maths teacher whom he feels has been unfairly targeting him for criticism. He asks you for advice on what he should do.

Please rate how appropriate the following responses are:

1. Sit down and talk to your friend to find out more about the reasons why his teacher may be unhappy with him.

    A.   A very appropriate thing to do

    B.   Appropriate, but not ideal

    C.   Inappropriate, but not awful

    D.   A very inappropriate thing to do

2. Tell your friend to go to the maths tutor and ask him why he has an issue with him.

    A.   A very appropriate thing to do

    B.   Appropriate, but not ideal

C. Inappropriate, but not awful

D. A very inappropriate thing to do

3. Tell your friend to ignore the issue and just continue to work as hard as possible in lessons.

A. A very appropriate thing to do

B. Appropriate, but not ideal

C. Inappropriate, but not awful

D. A very inappropriate thing to do

4. Mention the problem to your form tutor and ask for her advice on how to proceed.

A. A very appropriate thing to do

B. Appropriate, but not ideal

C. Inappropriate, but not awful

D. A very inappropriate thing to do

Example Scenario 2: Answers and Explanations

Question 1: A. A very appropriate thing to do

In this scenario it is important for you to know more about the situation, as it will help give you a better viewpoint from which to advise your friend. Additionally, discussing the issue may benefit your friend and help him realise why the problems are arising.

Question 2: D. A very inappropriate thing to do

This response would likely result in a discussion of a hostile nature and raise the level of conflict. It can also be viewed as a very confrontational response, which should always be avoided where possible – be it in school, work or as part of a team.

Question 3: C. Inappropriate, but not awful

While it would certainly be advisable to work as hard as possible, this response fails to deal with the issue at hand. The problem would go unresolved. Although avoiding conflict this is a temporary solution that may lead to the issue resurfacing at a later date.

Question 4: A. A very appropriate thing to do

This would be a very appropriate way of directly addressing the issue in a mature, non-confrontational manner. Form tutors are there to help with these types of issues, and throughout your medical career you will have supervisors there to help you when required.

Communication Skills

Many scenarios in SJT focus on communication skills, from dealing with angry or upset individuals to conflict resolution and even breaking bad news. They are not just testing your intellectual ability but also your emotional maturity. In addition to verbal communication, it is important to consider the non-verbal communication aspects of a scenario. For instance, a scenario might tell you someone 'looks upset'. This is a form of non-verbal communication that needs to be considered, as it demonstrates a person's emotional state.

When deciding on answers there are numerous factors to consider. Answers that express ideas clearly and sensitively are far more likely to be positive overall. It is equally important to consider the place in which the discussions take place. Consider the following scenario:

You are the passenger in a car being driven by your mother when her phone rings. You answer on her behalf only to find out that your grandfather has just passed away.

How appropriate is the following?

You immediately inform your mother so she can turn around and head straight to the hospital.

On the one hand, it seems that this may be an appropriate response as you should obviously inform her about what's happened. However, you must consider the time and place. Is it appropriate to break bad news while someone is driving? This is obviously a risk not just to you and your mother, but also to all other road users. She will immediately become distracted and this may even lead to a crash.

The answer here is 'a very inappropriate thing to do'. Based on the decision to break bad news in inappropriate surroundings you would be creating a risk to your mother and yourself, as well as other road users. It is vital that, in addition to communicating clearly and sensitively, you always consider the appropriate surroundings and best place to do so.

Some actions include seeking help or advice from others (example Scenario 2, Question 4). You will often be presented with scenarios outside your comfort zone, which you have not previously encountered. Seeking advice from someone more experienced is a very positive action, as it shows maturity and demonstrates that you know your limits.

> **Top Tip:** Although seeking advice is positive, be careful that the action doesn't involve you passing off your problems onto someone else. This would be a negative action as you fail to address the problem at hand.

In all communication-based questions, ensure you are always within your remit. Common questions focus on scenarios such as the following:

You are a medical student shadowing a GP when she gets called out of the room halfway through a consultation. The patient looks at you and asks you for their test results.

It is crucial you always remember who you are in each scenario (the introduction will tell you). You need to base your responses on what you should be doing at that level. Clearly, in the scenario above, it would be very inappropriate for you as the medical student to release any test results to the patient.

Example Scenario 3

> You are a junior doctor, having just started your first placement on an infectious diseases ward, when you notice that one of the senior nurses has been constantly forgetting to put on a protective apron when going into high risk patients' rooms. You recall how important this is from previous lectures but also know that this nurse is in charge of providing feedback on your performance to your consultant.

Please rate how important each of the following are:

1. As the senior nurse has far more healthcare experience you decide to ignore it.

    A.   Very Important

    B.   Important

    C.   Of minor importance

    D.   Not important at all

2. Mention the finding to your consultant at your next meeting.

    A.   Very important

    B.   Important

    C.   Of minor importance

    D.   Not important at all

3. Mention to the nurse your observation and how important wearing aprons are.

    A.   Very important

    B.   Important

    C.   Of minor importance

    D.   Not important at all

4. Continue to monitor it as you are hesitant to make a bad impression on a respected senior staff member.

    A.   Very important

    B.   Important

    C.   Of minor importance

    D.   Not important at all

Example Scenario 3: Answers and Explanations

Question 1: D. Not important at all

In this instance, the fact that she has more experience than you is neither the most important thing nor a mitigating factor. What is crucial is that, without your intervention, there is a risk to patient safety. So, while respecting the experience of senior colleagues is crucial, this response is far from ideal given the situation.

Question 2: C. Of minor importance

While recognising a need to act, this particular response is not particularly important as the same end goal can be achieved but without the need to involve your consultant. Generally, only the most pressing concerns should be reserved for your consultant.

Question 3: A. Very important

This is crucial in this situation. It rectifies an issue that has the potential to endanger patient safety, while also treating a senior employee with respect. The ability to discuss important issues with colleagues in a mature and non-confrontational manner is essential in medicine.

Question 4: D. Not important at all

Again, the most important thing is patient safety. Failure to mention the issue or intervene is poor medical practice and is 'hiding' from the problem. This highlights how little importance this response carries.

Integrity, Professionalism and Probity

Integrity, professionalism and probity are key buzzwords used in medicine. As a doctor, you are expected to act as a professional, maintaining professional standards both in and out of work. These include:

- Acting with integrity
- Acting in ways that promote and maintain the public trust for the medical profession
- Taking responsibility
- Keeping up to date and providing the highest standards of care
- Admitting when you are wrong and reflecting on events

Many SJT scenarios are designed to push you on these issues. Answers that compromise your integrity and trustworthiness are always going to be negative. This includes:

- Not addressing the problems at hand in order to avoid conflict
- Actions that are illegal or violate basic confidentiality
- Any form of dishonest behaviour

Although it seems obvious that dishonest actions will be negative, SJTs can still create scenarios whereby this choice becomes difficult. Withholding information from someone is obviously negative. But what if it is done with their best interests at heart? Is it right to withhold certain details of someone's death in order to spare the feelings of their relatives? The simple answer, for the purposes of SJT, is no. Never withhold any information just because you want to spare someone's feelings. People have a right to know details, should they wish. Often, knowing what's happened will help with the grieving process.

Confidentiality

Confidentiality is a complicated area far above the level required for the UKCAT exam. There have, however, been questions which require a basic understanding of confidentiality in previous exams.

The purpose of confidentiality is that it allows patients and doctors to form a bond with trust. Patients feel free to disclose personal information, often essential for making the correct diagnosis, knowing that it will stay between them and the doctor. For the purposes of SJT you must respect this right. Any answers that involve distributing or sharing patient information with others is usually negative.

Although there are several instances when you may break confidentiality, for the purposes of UKCAT the simple rule is that unless a person's life is at risk, you do not break confidentiality. If a patient has told you something which they do not want their doctor to know, then you should encourage them to allow you to tell their doctor by clearly explaining the importance.

Example Scenario 4

> You are the captain of your sixth form football team and a teammate approaches you saying that the team's results have not been good of late and that he feels you should consider stepping down as captain. You have, however, been enjoying the role of captain and would like to continue.

Please rate how appropriate the following responses are:

1. Step down as captain immediately to avoid conflict.

    A.   A very appropriate thing to do

    B.   Appropriate, but not ideal

    C.   Inappropriate, but not awful

    D.   A very inappropriate thing to do

2. Discuss with your teammate any issues he has with your captaincy and tell him you'll take them on board to improve.

    A.   A very appropriate thing to do

    B.   Appropriate, but not ideal

C.   Inappropriate, but not awful

D.   A very inappropriate thing to do

3. Call a team meeting telling your team the views of your teammate and ask for their opinion.

A.   A very appropriate thing to do

B.   Appropriate, but not ideal

C.   Inappropriate, but not awful

D.   A very inappropriate thing to do

4. You immediately tell your teammate you will not be stepping down but you appreciate his views and will work hard to address the issues he raised.

A.   A very appropriate thing to do

B.   Appropriate, but not ideal

C.   Inappropriate, but not awful

D.   A very inappropriate thing to do

Example Scenario 4: Answers and Explanations

Question 1: D. A very inappropriate thing to do

As you go through your medical career you will constantly encounter challenges. Stepping down at the first sign of difficulty is not the ideal way to approach things. While stepping down may ultimately be correct, it would be advisable to discuss things further first in order to make an informed decision.

Question 2: A. A very appropriate thing to do

This is a non-confrontational and mature way to approach the situation. It takes into account the concerns of your teammate and gives you the time to come to a measured and well thought out decision.

Question 3: C. Inappropriate, but not awful

While it is often important to consult the opinions of others, it is very possible your teammate came to you in confidence and would rather his views be kept between the two of you. It would likely be wiser to consult the opinions of one or two senior teammates in a more private manner before addressing the whole team. Furthermore, this action may create a situation whereby people are forced to take sides, increasing the chances of conflict.

Question 4: B. Appropriate, but not ideal

In this scenario you are within your rights to continue as captain. It also admirable that you wish to rectify any issues your teammate has brought up. However, immediately refusing to even consider stepping down may be construed as very stubborn and uncooperative.

Teamwork and Leadership

Teamwork questions in SJT often focus on testing your understanding of the roles of team members and leaders, in combination with communication skills. Frequently these communication skills will revolve around conflict resolution, where team members disagree with each other, or with a leader.

It is important to remember that all teams need structure and leadership. The role of the leader is to ensure the smooth running of the team, in order to achieve its task. To do this, the team leader must be prepared to listen to team members and involve relevant team members when making decisions. This is a two-way line of communication. Listening is essential. Not only does it ensure decisions are discussed and more likely to be correct; it also makes the team members feel valued and appreciated, boosting the morale and productivity of the team.

In SJT scenarios where you are leading a team, it is therefore essential that you consider answers which involve you listening to, and taking feedback from, your team members. You will need to ensure workload is shared evenly across team members and that people are undertaking the tasks to which they are best suited. There must always be a clear, two-way line of communication.

Example Scenario 5

You are in your final year of medical school. As you near a set of important exams, one of your friends is beginning to become withdrawn and is showing signs of struggling with increased stress levels.

Please rate how important the following are:

1. Immediately tell a staff member about your friend in order to quickly deal with the problem.

    A.   Very Important

    B.   Important

    C.   Of minor importance

    D.   Not important at all

2. Discuss the situation with your other friends to see if you can come up with a solution together.

    A.   Very Important

    B.   Important

    C.   Of minor importance

    D.   Not important at all

3. Talk to your friend to find out if anything is bothering them and offer any help you can give them.

   A.   Very Important

   B.   Important

   C.   Of minor importance

   D.   Not important at all

4. Keep your distance from them for fear you could exacerbate the situation.

   A.   Very Important

   B.   Important

   C.   Of minor importance

   D.   Not important at all

Example Scenario 5: Answers and Explanations

Question 1: D. Not important at all

It would not be advisable to bypass your friend by going straight to a member of staff. Your friend could react negatively and become more likely to conceal any underlying issues they have.

Question 2: C. Of minor importance

It would be better to start by talking to your friend, finding out more information about what's going on. By widening the number of people involved it could complicate an already complex and delicate matter.

Question 3: A. Very important

By doing this you are addressing the problem at hand and showing concern for your friend, while not threatening to get over-involved. As a result, your friend will be more likely to confide in you as they know you have their best interests at heart.

Question 4: D. Not important at all

This action, or lack thereof, may lead to problems snowballing, as your friend becomes even more withdrawn and feels that there is nobody they can talk to. It is important to demonstrate your emotional maturity and to be supportive, letting your friend know you are there to help him.

Pressure and Prioritisation

Pressure and prioritisation are intrinsically linked concepts. The more pressured you are, the more essential it becomes that you prioritise your tasks to ensure that the most important ones are completed. Pressure can be divided into 'acute' and 'chronic' pressure.

Acute pressure encompasses situations where there is a sudden event that puts people under pressure. This is often the result of unpredictable events and emergencies. SJT scenarios involving acute pressure often focus on work as a junior doctor, where you are suddenly faced with a large number of tasks, all of which seemingly need to be completed immediately. When choosing answers for scenarios involving acute pressure, look for those that organise and prioritise the tasks, so that urgent and important (see below) ones are completed first. If you're struggling, options which involve seeking help from colleagues or seniors are nearly always positive.

Chronic pressure tends to be the result of numerous long-term tasks that all require significant time devotion. This may take the form of revision for exams, commitment to sports teams etc. To select suitable answer options for these questions, it is essential to look for options that break tasks into manageable steps (e.g. creating revision timetables and allocating realistic, regular time devotion). They should set realistic goals and demonstrate perseverance.

> **Top Tip:** If you are presented with a scenario where you are struggling, look for answer options that incorporate seeking help and advice from colleagues and seniors. !

When deciding how to prioritise tasks you can consider dividing them into those which are important/not important and urgent/non-urgent:

	Urgent	**Non-Urgent**
Important	Category I	Category II
Not Important	Category III	Category IV

Category I tasks are both urgent and important. This might be calling an ambulance if someone has collapsed or leaving a burning building. These are tasks to which you must always allocate the highest priority (very appropriate/very important). They always trump other tasks.

Category II tasks include those that are important but not urgent, i.e. those that require regular time devotion, such as revision or exercise. Category III tasks are the quick interruptions in life, such as answering a phone call. Category IV tasks include those which are neither important nor urgent, and which should always be given the lowest priority. These might include watching TV, playing computer games etc.

Time for some practice! Try answering the following **20 Practice Scenarios** containing **67 questions**. There is a mixture of 'appropriateness' and 'importance' style questions. You have 26 minutes to answer all questions. Detailed explanations are provided. Good luck!

Practice Sets

Question Scenario 1

You are a work experience student on a ward round. You have just witnessed your consultant inform a patient that they have a form of lung cancer. Shortly after, you run into the patient's daughter, who was not present, and she asks you how her mother is doing.

Please rate how appropriate the following responses are:

1. Inform the patient's daughter you have not heard any news recently on her mother's progress.

    A. A very appropriate thing to do

    B. Appropriate, but not ideal

    C. Inappropriate, but not awful

    D. A very inappropriate thing to do

2. Inform the patient's daughter that she has just been diagnosed with a form of lung cancer.

    A. A very appropriate thing to do

    B. Appropriate, but not ideal

    C. Inappropriate, but not awful

    D. A very inappropriate thing to do

3. Tell the patient's daughter this is information you are unable to give.

    A. A very appropriate thing to do

    B. Appropriate, but not ideal

    C. Inappropriate, but not awful

    D. A very inappropriate thing to do

4. After explaining that this is information you are unable to give, offer to speak to the consultant and arrange for him to come and have a discussion with the patient's daughter.

    A. A very appropriate thing to do

    B. Appropriate, but not ideal

    C. Inappropriate, but not awful

    D. A very inappropriate thing to do

Question Scenario 2

You are a junior doctor on a urology rotation. You find that due to short inpatient stays you have a lot of free time on a daily basis where you have no jobs or patients to attend to.

Please rate how appropriate the following responses are:

1. Offer to help other junior doctors on busier wards.

    A. A very appropriate thing to do

    B. Appropriate, but not ideal

   C. Inappropriate, but not awful

   D. A very inappropriate thing to do

2. Ask your consultant to schedule extra outpatient sessions for you.

   A. A very appropriate thing to do

   B. Appropriate, but not ideal

   C. Inappropriate, but not awful

   D. A very inappropriate thing to do

3. Mention the free time to your educational supervisor and ask her advice.

   A. A very appropriate thing to do

   B. Appropriate, but not ideal

   C. Inappropriate, but not awful

   D. A very inappropriate thing to do

Question Scenario 3

You are a junior doctor on a cardiology rotation with one other partner. When it comes to dividing jobs you find that he always goes for the easy and quick jobs leaving you the harder jobs. Despite this you usually finish your jobs at the same time.

Please rate how important each of the following are:

1. Mention to your supervisor that your partner is being unfair.

   A. Very important

   B. Important

   C. Of minor importance

   D. Not important at all

2. Discuss with your partner that you have noticed this pattern.

   A. Very important

   B. Important

   C. Of minor importance

   D. Not important at all

3. Ignore the situation to avoid starting a conflict.

   A. Very important

   B. Important

   C. Of minor importance

   D. Not important at all

Question Scenario 4

While buying a sandwich at your local supermarket you receive £50 change when in reality you should have received £5 change. You only notice this when you are at the bus stop five minutes away from the shop.

Please rate how important each of the following are:

1. Make a note of the error and return the excess change tomorrow when you return to the supermarket.

    A. Very important

    B. Important

    C. Of minor importance

    D. Not important at all

2. Keep hold of the change for the time being but do not spend it.

    A. Very important

    B. Important

    C. Of minor importance

    D. Not important at all

3. Return immediately to the shop and hand back the £50 for the correct change.

    A. Very important

    B. Important

    C. Of minor importance

    D. Not important at all

Question Scenario 5

You are the junior doctor on the cardiology ward and a pharmacist approaches you saying that the dosage of a certain drug for a patient has been halved by your consultant. The pharmacist says he has rarely seen this dosage used and asks you why but you are not sure and your consultant is not on the ward.

Please rate how appropriate the following responses are:

1. Change the dosage back to the normal amount.

    A. A very appropriate thing to do

    B. Appropriate, but not ideal

    C. Inappropriate, but not awful

    D. A very inappropriate thing to do

2. Offer to phone your consultant and get back to the pharmacist as soon as possible.

    A. A very appropriate thing to do

    B. Appropriate, but not ideal

    C. Inappropriate, but not awful

    D. A very inappropriate thing to do

3. Your consultant is very experienced and knowledgeable so decide to keep the dose unchanged.

   A. A very appropriate thing to do

   B. Appropriate, but not ideal

   C. Inappropriate, but not awful

   D. A very inappropriate thing to do

Question Scenario 6

You are walking home after an evening shift when you witness a car crash into a parked car outside a house, causing minor damage to both vehicles. The driver, who appears unhurt, speeds off into the distance but you are able to note his license plate number.

Please rate how important each of the following are:

1. Immediately call 999 to report the car crash

   A. Very important

   B. Important

   C. Of minor importance

   D. Not important at all

2. Continue on your way home as nobody was injured.

   A. Very important

   B. Important

   C. Of minor importance

   D. Not important at all

3. Knock on the house of the owners of the parked car and inform them of what you saw and the license plate number.

   A. Very important

   B. Important

   C. Of minor importance

   D. Not important at all

Question Scenario 7

You are working a weekend job as a shop assistant and you spot a good friend attempting to steal a pair of jeans from the display. You know that your friend's family has had money troubles recently and he has never done anything like this before.

Please rate how appropriate the following responses are:

1. As you sympathise with your friend's situation, pretend not to see him.

   A. A very appropriate thing to do

   B. Appropriate, but not ideal

C. Inappropriate, but not awful

D. A very inappropriate thing to do

2. Rush over to your friend and tell him to put the jeans back and offer to speak to him after your shift.

A. A very appropriate thing to do

B. Appropriate, but not idea

C. Inappropriate, but not awful

D. A very inappropriate thing to do

3. Alert your store supervisor to the attempted theft but explain he is your friend and that this is out of character for him.

A. A very appropriate thing to do

B. Appropriate, but not ideal

C. Inappropriate, but not awful

D. A very inappropriate thing to do

Question Scenario 8

You are a medical student on a surgical ward. You have a very important football game for the medical school that you cannot be late for. The time for the football game is also specifically set in your timetable. The ward is swamped with work and, as you are about to leave, the consultant asks if you would not mind staying behind a couple of hours extra to help.

Please rate how appropriate the following responses are:

1. Agree to stay and help your consultant, missing the match.

A. A very appropriate thing to do

B. Appropriate, but not ideal

C. Inappropriate, but not awful

D. A very inappropriate thing to do

2. Inform the consultant you are unable to stay due to an important prior engagement.

A. A very appropriate thing to do

B. Appropriate, but not ideal

C. Inappropriate, but not awful

D. A very inappropriate thing to do

3. Inform the consultant you are unable to stay but offer to help stay later tomorrow if required as you will be free that afternoon.

A. A very appropriate thing to do

B. Appropriate, but not ideal

C. Inappropriate, but not awful

D. A very inappropriate thing to do

Question Scenario 9

You are preparing for an important two-person A-level presentation to be given later this morning when your partner rings you to say she will be unable to attend as she is unwell. However, on a social media site, photos of her at a party from last night have been posted moments ago.

Please rate how important each of the following are:

1. Suggest to your colleague she immediately removes the photos from the website.

    A. Very important

    B. Important

    C. Of minor importance

    D. Not important at all

2. Find out what's happened and in what way she is unwell.

    A. Very important

    B. Important

    C. Of minor importance

    D. Not important at all

3. Ask a fellow student for advice on how to proceed as you are unsure.

    A. Very important

    B. Important

    C. Of minor importance

    D. Not important at all

4. Inform your teacher that your partner is has rung in sick despite attending a party the previous day.

    A. Very important

    B. Important

    C. Of minor importance

    D. Not important at all

Question Scenario 10

You have just been set a very tough but important essay in your AS-level economics class and you are finding it very difficult to prepare for it. A friend in the year above remarks that he did the same essay last year and did very well. He asks if you would like to see the essay.

Please rate how appropriate the following responses are:

1. Thank your friend for the offer but instead ask if he could spend an hour teaching you some key points.

    A. A very appropriate thing to do

    B. Appropriate, but not ideal

C. Inappropriate, but not awful

D. A very inappropriate thing to do

2. Accept the copy of the essay and memorise just a few of the key points to use in your essay.

A. A very appropriate thing to do

B. Appropriate, but not ideal

C. Inappropriate, but not awful

D. A very inappropriate thing to do

3. Decline the offer and continue to prepare for the essay as you were before.

A. A very appropriate thing to do

B. Appropriate, but not ideal

C. Inappropriate, but not awful

D. A very inappropriate thing to do

Question Scenario 11

You are the junior doctor sent to take blood from an elderly patient who previously had leukaemia. From the initial results in the notes you can see it is highly likely there has been a recurrence of leukaemia but not all the tests have been completed. The patient asks has his leukaemia come back.

Please rate how appropriate the following responses are:

1. Explain to the patient that you don't have all his results but will speak to him once you do.

A. A very appropriate thing to do

B. Appropriate, but not ideal

C. Inappropriate, but not awful

D. A very inappropriate thing to do

2. Inform the patient that the leukaemia has most likely returned but the tests are yet to be finished.

A. A very appropriate thing to do

B. Appropriate, but not ideal

C. Inappropriate, but not awful

D. A very inappropriate thing to do

3. Inform the patient the leukaemia has not returned.

A. A very appropriate thing to do

B. Appropriate, but not ideal

C. Inappropriate, but not awful

D. A very inappropriate thing to do

4. Explain to the patient that you don't have all the results yet but once you do will ask a senior member of the team to come and speak with him.

   A. A very appropriate thing to do

   B. Appropriate, but not ideal

   C. Inappropriate, but not awful

   D. A very inappropriate thing to do

Question Scenario 12

You are volunteering at your local elderly care home on a Saturday afternoon. What started as a friendly discussion between two residents has become confrontational and threatens to turn physical.

Please rate how important the following are:

1. Try to talk to the residents and resolve the situation by yourself.

   A. Very important

   B. Important

   C. Of minor importance

   D. Not important at all

2. Call upon a nearby staff nurse to help diffuse the situation.

   A. Very important

   B. Important

   C. Of minor importance

   D. Not important at all

3. After the incident is dealt with, encourage the two residents to spend more time with each other to work out their differences.

   A. Very Important

   B. Important

   C. Of minor importance

   D. Not important at all

Question Scenario 13

You are on your way home after a busy day and you get off the tube platform. At the far end of the platform you see a blind man struggling to navigate his way around and there appears to be no tube staff nearby.

Please rate how appropriate the following responses are:

1. Wait to see if one of the fellow commuters helps him.

   A. A very appropriate thing to do

   B. Appropriate, but not ideal

C. Inappropriate, but not awful

D. A very inappropriate thing to do

2. Go and find the nearest member of staff and alert them that there is a blind passenger who requires assistance.

A. A very appropriate thing to do

B. Appropriate, but not ideal

C. Inappropriate, but not awful

D. A very inappropriate thing to do

3. Head over to assist the blind commuter as best you can.

A. A very appropriate thing to do

B. Appropriate, but not ideal

C. Inappropriate, but not awful

D. A very inappropriate thing to do

4. As it has been a long day, head home in the hope that a staff member or another commuter will go to help.

A. A very appropriate thing to do

B. Appropriate, but not ideal

C. Inappropriate, but not awful

D. A very inappropriate thing to do

Question Scenario 14

A mother and her teenage son come to see you while you are working as a junior doctor in a general practice. She is very concerned and angry about an apparent change in his behaviour and can be heard arguing with him in the waiting room. The mother does most of the talking, while the teenager appears subdued and uncomfortable talking in front of his mother.

Please rate how important the following are:

1. Try to get the son to talk more about his side of the story.

A. Very important

B. Important

C. Of minor importance

D. Not important at all

2. Tell the mother to stay quiet as she is affecting her son's ability to speak.

A. Very important

B. Important

C. Of minor importance

D. Not important at all

3. Ask the mother and son if they want to talk separately in order to make them feel more comfortable.

    A. Very important

    B. Important

    C. Of minor importance

    D. Not important at all

Question Scenario 15

You are a junior doctor on a ward round and realise that you have mixed up the first two patients' notes and so have been documenting the findings in the incorrect notes. You are still midway through the busy ward round but know you need to correct your error.

Please rate how appropriate the following responses are:

1. Inform the consultant of your error and let him know you will correct it right away.

    A. A very appropriate thing to do

    B. Appropriate, but not ideal

    C. Inappropriate, but not awful

    D. A very inappropriate thing to do

2. Wait until after the ward round finishes and quickly correct the notes.

    A. A very appropriate thing to do

    B. Appropriate, but not ideal

    C. Inappropriate, but not awful

    D. A very inappropriate thing to do

3. Ask the other junior doctor on the ward round for advice on what to do.

    A. A very appropriate thing to do

    B. Appropriate, but not ideal

    C. Inappropriate, but not awful

    D. A very inappropriate thing to do

Question Scenario 16

You and your colleague are both doctors. During a visit to your colleague's apartment you see he is taking controlled medication obtained through falsified prescriptions. As well as this, you suspect his addiction is beginning to spiral out of control.

Please rate how important the following are:

1. Talk to your colleague to ask why he is taking the medication.

    A. Very important

    B. Important

C. Of minor importance

D. Not important at all

2. Report your colleague to your consultant because he is possibly abusing patient supplies.

    A. Very important

    B. Important

    C. Of minor importance

    D. Not important at all

3. Try to cover for your colleague when he makes errors at work.

    A. Very important

    B. Important

    C. Of minor importance

    D. Not important at all

4. Offer support and encourage your colleague to seek help as soon as possible.

    A. Very important

    B. Important

    C. Of minor importance

    D. Not important at all

Question Scenario 17

You are working as an FY1 doctor in an accident and emergency department. You see a patient and diagnose them with an illness, which requires a complex treatment. You decide on a treatment; however, your FY1 colleague and a nurse disagree with your plan.

Please rate how important the following are:

1. Have a discussion with the nurse and your colleague in order to understand why they disagree with your choice.

    A. Very important

    B. Important

    C. Of minor importance

    D. Not important at all

2. After a brief discussion with the nurse and your colleague you disagree with their opinion and go ahead with your original decision.

    A. Very important

    B. Important

    C. Of minor importance

    D. Not important at all

3. Go against your own decision on the recommendation of the nurse and your colleague.

   A. Very important

   B. Important

   C. Of minor importance

   D. Not important at all

4. Consult a senior doctor about the case to get their advice.

   A. Very important

   B. Important

   C. Of minor importance

   D. Not important at all

Question Scenario 18

You are the junior doctor on a ward round where you observe a consultant gaining consent from the family of a seriously ill patient for organ donation. The family, although seemingly reluctant, eventually agree. You bump into the family alone shortly after and they tell you they felt pressured and really would not like to agree to organ donation.

Please rate how appropriate the following responses are:

1. Tell the family to take the issue up with the consultant directly as due to your level you are unable to help.

   A. A very appropriate thing to do

   B. Appropriate, but not ideal

   C. Inappropriate, but not awful

   D. A very inappropriate thing to do

2. Tell the family you will let the consultant know about their concerns and ask him to speak to them again.

   A. A very appropriate thing to do

   B. Appropriate, but not ideal

   C. Inappropriate, but not awful

   D. A very inappropriate thing to do

3. Explore the family's concerns and answer any questions you can that they have regarding organ donation.

   A. A very appropriate thing to do

   B. Appropriate, but not ideal

   C. Inappropriate, but not awful

   D. A very inappropriate thing to do

4. Inform your registrar (senior doctor) of the problem as it is likely she is well equipped to deal with the situation.

   A. A very appropriate thing to do

   B. Appropriate, but not ideal

   C. Inappropriate, but not awful

   D. A very inappropriate thing to do

Question Scenario 19

As one of the school prefects you are on patrol around the school. During the patrol you notice a younger boy is being picked on by some of his peers.

Please rate how important the following are:

1. Allow the young boy to fight back against the bullies.

   A. Very important

   B. Important

   C. Of minor importance

   D. Not important at all

2. Break up the situation and start antagonising the bullies so that they understand how it feels.

   A. Very important

   B. Important

   C. Of minor importance

   D. Not important at all

3. Reassure the boy who was picked on that he has nothing to worry about.

   A. Very important

   B. Important

   C. Of minor importance

   D. Not important at all

Question Scenario 20

You are in a rush on the way to the station to catch a train you are running late for. On your way you notice a wallet on the ground with a name and address tag on it. Stopping even for one minute will mean you miss your train and will be late for the concert you are planning to attend.

Please rate how appropriate the following responses are:

1. Pick up the wallet and take it with you and return it to the police station after the concert.

   A. A very appropriate thing to do

   B. Appropriate, but not ideal

C. Inappropriate, but not awful

D. A very inappropriate thing to do

2. As the concert tickets were very expensive and you do not want to miss it, rush by and ignore the wallet.

A. A very appropriate thing to do

B. Appropriate, but not ideal

C. Inappropriate, but not awful

D. A very inappropriate thing to do

3. Stop to pick up the wallet and hand it to a good friend, instructing them to hand it in to the police station.

A. A very appropriate thing to do

B. Appropriate, but not ideal

C. Inappropriate, but not awful

D. A very inappropriate thing to do

Answers

Scenario 1

Question 1: D. A very inappropriate thing to do

This is highly inappropriate as this response is essentially lying to the patient's family, which is never acceptable. While it is a very sensitive situation, it is crucial to remain honest while respecting confidentiality and not overstepping the responsibilities of your role.

Question 2: D. A very inappropriate thing to do

This is also very inappropriate because, as a work experience student, this is information you are not qualified to be giving. Furthermore, it is highly likely you will not know enough about the patient or the condition to answer the follow-up questions. It is crucial in medicine to know the limitations of your role and know when to contact a senior.

Question 3: B. Appropriate, but not ideal

While this is honest and respecting the limitations of the medical student role it is somewhat insensitive and does not get the patient's daughter any closer to finding out what is happening with her mother. It fails to resolve the situation.

Question 4: A. A very appropriate thing to do

This is the textbook response as it does not involve anything outside of the remit of a work experience student's duties and is also proactive in trying to find a solution to this sensitive situation. It also involves good communication skills in order to relay the information in a sensible manner.

Scenario 2

Question 1: B. Appropriate, but not ideal

Although this response is very well meaning, you are attached to a specific rotation for a reason and thus you should attempt to re-invest your time in a manner that will help your specific team. However, it is far from an unreasonable action.

Question 2: A. A very appropriate thing to do

This is an ideal response as it is pro-active and shows your consultant you are eager to help in any way possible. It also will help out your urology team in outpatients, making the schedule run more efficiently.

Question 3: A. A very appropriate thing to do

This is again a very appropriate response as your supervisors are in place to assist you with such issues. It will also highlight an issue that can be addressed for future junior doctors on your rotation, thus improving their future work environment.

Scenario 3

Question 1: C. Of minor importance

In a situation such as this, it is advisable to deal directly with the person involved and tackle the issue head on. Involving a third party is not important or necessary at this stage. If you were to speak to your partner and he was still refusing to take into account your concerns then this may be an important step. However, if you felt your partner to be intimidating or unapproachable this may be considered.

Question 2: A. Very important

This is the most important step to take in this situation. The discussion should be in a mature and non-argumentative manner. It is important to get the viewpoint of your partner as it may be possible he is unaware of his behaviour. Also the fact that you finish your jobs at the same time means your partner may be struggling to complete even basic jobs and may need further help.

Question 3: D. Not important at all

Although generally speaking, conflict should always be avoided where possible, in this instance it is far more important to discuss this issue that has arisen. As mentioned earlier this should obviously be done in as mature and non-confrontational a way as possible.

Scenario 4

Question 1: B. Important

While the ideal response would be to turn back immediately this action crucially has the correct intention of returning money to the rightful place after an honest oversight by both parties.

Question 2: D. Not important at all

This is not an important action and is very non-committal. It fails to show a strong intention to return the money and deciding not to spend the money in the interim is a poor compromise.

Question 3: A. Very important

It is essential that if this error is recognised it is acted upon swiftly. This shows honesty and integrity, which are both crucial skills in the medical profession. It is also important to consider that this will ensure the store worker avoids repercussions that may have come their way had the money not been returned.

Scenario 5

Question 1: D. A very inappropriate thing to do

It would be risky and somewhat irresponsible behaviour to just assume an error has been made and change the dosage back to normal. In this scenario attempts should be made to definitively find out why the dose was changed.

Question 2: A. A very appropriate thing to do

This is the ideal response as not only does it resolve the issue at hand but it is using your own initiative and taking responsibility for the situation, which is always a great thing to do in all aspects of life.

Question 3: D. A very inappropriate thing to do

Just assuming that the dose is correct or incorrect is very dangerous and compromises patient safety. Even the most experienced clinicians are capable of making dosing errors so it would be wise to double check with the consultant as quickly as possible.

Scenario 6

Question 1: B. Important

In the event of witnessing a car crash it is important to contact the police, particularly if you have important information or were the only witness of the accident. As no one has been injured it would be more appropriate to contact 111 as 999 should be reserved for potentially life-threatening emergencies.

Question 2: D. Not important at all

This is not an important action in the situation and achieves nothing. While it is good that nobody was seriously hurt there are still several important steps that must be taken to ensure the relevant people receive the necessary information.

Question 3: A. Very important

This is very important to do as it is likely that, without your intervention, the owners of the car will be unaware of what has occurred. If you imagine yourself in such a situation, it is highly likely you would wish to know if it had been your car involved in such an incident.

Scenario 7

Question 1: D. A very inappropriate thing to do

While it is natural to feel sorry for your friend, as an employee of the shop, it is your duty to act in an appropriate manner to ensure the theft does not occur. Ignoring a problem is never a good solution.

Question 2: B. Appropriate, but not ideal

This response addresses the issue directly and also offers to help out the friend by speaking to him after the shift as well as helping him avoid the trouble he would have got himself in. However, as a member of the shop, it is important to follow shop protocol and not to act with double standards just because it is a friend. The same principles apply in a medical career.

Question 3: A. A very appropriate thing to do

This response addresses the situation and involves correct escalation to the appropriate senior with provision of accurate information with background information that the supervisor can choose to use as they require.

Scenario 8

Question 1: C. Inappropriate, but not awful

While it is admirable to want to stay behind and help it would be letting down all your team-mates if you miss the game. Furthermore, work–life balance is crucial and, as long as you are fulfilling the duties of your role and not compromising patient safety, you are within your rights to attend the game. Although generally speaking it is always ideal for medical students to help out any way they can.

Question 2: A. A very appropriate thing to do

This, although failing to help with the situation on the ward, is a very appropriate thing to do in this situation, especially as the time slot for the football game is specifically designated in your timetable.

Question 3: A. A very appropriate thing to do

This is also a very appropriate response; while still rightfully attending the football game, this response also shows initiative in offering to help at a later date, endearing yourself to your consultant in the process.

Scenario 9

Question 1: C. Of minor importance

While ultimately good advice, in this scenario, with the presentation a matter of hours away, this is not the most important response. It does not solve the issue of why your partner is away or come up with a solution for how to proceed with the presentation.

Question 2: A. Very important

It is crucial not to jump to conclusions as it is possible that, for instance, your partner may have had a case of food poisoning from food at the party. Also, as they are your partner for an important presentation it is crucial that you maintain good communication skills and trust throughout.

Question 3: B. Important

If you are unsure, it is important to seek advice from an appropriate source. In this instance a peer is very much an appropriate person to ask. However, if you feel you are able to proceed alone, it is certainly not essential to consult the advice of a peer, particularly in situations such as this one where the best course of action is to discuss the issue directly with the person in question.

Question 4: D. Not important at all

It is crucial not to make assumptions and jump to conclusions. It is neither essential nor advisable to inform your teacher that your colleague was at a party the night before, especially as you haven't even discussed this with your colleague.

Scenario 10

Question 1: A. A very appropriate thing to do

This is a constructive way to use your friend's help and does not run any risk of plagiarism. This would be a very appropriate suggestion.

Question 2: D. A very inappropriate thing to do

While this may seem like it will help you achieve a higher grade this is dishonest and is blatant plagiarism. It shows a lack of integrity that is undesirable for a career in medicine.

Question 3: B. Appropriate, but not ideal

While this is undoubtedly an honest approach it doesn't utilise the potential great learning resource that has been offered from your friend. Throughout your medical career it is important to seize all opportunities that help with your learning process.

Scenario 11

Question 1: B. Appropriate, but not ideal

While this response is both honest and adequately non-committal it is perhaps above a junior doctor's responsibility to be breaking news such as this. It would likely be more suitable to contact a senior doctor to do this.

Question 2: D. A very inappropriate thing to do

On occasions in medicine brutal honesty is not always the best approach and sometimes situations need to be handled in an honest but sensitive manner. Breaking the news to the patient in such a blunt manner and before the completion of all tests is highly inappropriate. You also need to remember that breaking news about a cancer diagnosis is outside the remit of a junior doctor.

Question 3: D. A very inappropriate thing to do

This is extremely dishonest and one of the worst possible things a doctor could say in such a situation. It is always crucial to keep integrity and the patient's feelings in mind when dealing with such difficult situations.

Question 4: A. A very appropriate thing to do

This is the most appropriate course of action as it maintains honesty and does not mislead the patient, while also offering to find the member of the team with the ideal experience to break the likely bad news to the patient.

Scenario 12

Question 1: C. Of minor importance

While action needs to be taken to deal with the situation, you are still relatively inexperienced and so it is more important to urgently inform the trained staff of what has just happened.

Question 2: A. Very important

It is very important to get the attention of an experienced professional who has been trained in dealing with these situations. The nurse will also be familiar with the residents, which increases the likelihood of successfully persuading the residents to keep calm.

Question 3: D, Not important at all

Although there are good intentions behind this act, it is possible that you could spark another argument between the residents, which is the last thing you would want to happen.

Scenario 13

Question 1: D. A very inappropriate thing to do

This is a very passive response and shows a lack of willingness to act and take responsibility for the situation. It is clear that the man is in need of help so it is important to act accordingly even if those around you are not.

Question 2: B. Appropriate, but not ideal

In this response you are somewhat active and use your initiative to contact the member of staff. However, it appears the man is in immediate need of help and may require attention sooner if possible.

Question 3: A. A very appropriate thing to do

This response brings immediate help to the gentleman in need and also involves taking ownership of the issue at hand. It is likely to be a relatively simple task of helping the commuter navigate and there is not necessarily a need to alert a member of staff.

Question 4: D. A very inappropriate thing to do

This is clearly an inappropriate response. It does not address the problem at hand and assuming that the man will be helped is dangerous. In such situations we should take it upon ourselves to help directly.

Scenario 14

Question 1: A. Very important

It seems that only one side is being heard. It may prove advantageous to listen to the teenager to see if he feels comfortable talking and explore what has been going on.

Question 2: D. Not important at all

This could further provoke the mother, which could further limit her son's desire to talk to you. The action is also quite confrontational and demonstrates poor communication skills.

Question 3: A. Very important

It appears that you are only hearing one side of the story and the teenager, for whatever reason, is not speaking up. It may be that he is reluctant to talk in front of his mother, so asking to speak to them alone may allow you to maintain trust, confidentiality and identify the underlying problem.

Scenario 15

Question 1: A. A very appropriate thing to do

This response involves taking accountability for your error and also demonstrating the honesty to admit to the relevant person you made an error. It is also crucial that the notes are amended as quickly as possible because another doctor or nurse may read the erroneous notes and, with this mistaken information, do something that may endanger the patient.

Question 2: D. A very inappropriate thing to do

This approach shows a lack of accountability and integrity and also endangers the patient's safety. Ward rounds can last for hours so it is imperative to correct the mistake as quickly as possible.

Question 3: A. A very appropriate thing to do

Remember the answers need not be complete – just because you ask for advice doesn't mean you won't also act quickly to resolve the situation. Seeking advice when unsure how to tackle a problem is an excellent skill looked for in doctors.

Scenario 16

Question 1: A. Very important

There could be many reasons behind his actions. So it is important to clarify why he is taking prescription medication before you take any further action.

Question 2: D. Not important at all

Going straight to the senior members may complicate matters and drive your colleague further into the use of medication. It would also weaken any bond you had with your colleague and make him feel more isolated. Remember, you do not have all of the facts yet and making allegations can have profound effects on his career.

Question 3: D. Not important at all

This action could eventually lead to serious consequences if your colleague proceeds to make continual errors and patient safety is seriously compromised. In addition, constantly covering for him will reduce your own work output and increase the chance you will make errors.

Question 4: A. Very important

By persuading him to tackle the problem straight away, you could start your colleague on the road to recovery. Knowing you are supporting him will help him realise his problems and improve his chances of success.

Scenario 17

Question 1: A. Very important

It is very important to discuss it with them because there may have been a key detail you over-looked or perhaps they overlooked. An open dialogue and discussion, especially when there may be disagreement, is essential among healthcare professionals and improves patient safety and outcomes.

Question 2: D. Not important at all

Since you are not a senior member it is not a good idea to overrule a clinical decision, especially when two people have expressed concerns. You should discuss the case with someone more senior before proceeding.

Question 3: D. Not important at all

Just because you are outnumbered it does not necessarily mean you are wrong. It is important to back yourself because it could be that you know something to be right but struggle to convince someone else. If in doubt you should discuss the plan with someone more senior first.

Question 4: A. Very important

When there is a conflict of opinions it is very important to discuss the issues with someone more experienced; in this case a senior doctor who can offer clinical advice.

Scenario 18

Question 1: D. A very inappropriate thing to do

This response fails to help the family and is also fairly insensitive as it involves refusing to help in a situation where you are able to do so. Also it is likely that the family will be somewhat daunted by the prospect of speaking to the consultant given the earlier events.

Question 2: A. A very appropriate thing to do

This is a good response and involves the use of communication skills to help resolve the issue. It also gives an opportunity to inform the consultant of the situation as he/she may not have been aware the first time round that the family were reluctant.

Question 3: A. A very appropriate thing to do

It is possible that the reason the family are reluctant is that they misunderstood some of the details the consultant was trying to convey. By exploring their concerns and answering any questions you are improving their understanding as well as gaining a better idea yourself of why this issue has arisen.

Question 4: C. Inappropriate, but not awful

In this situation it is better to refer the issue back to the person who took the consent in the first place, not a new person. Also, as the most senior member of the team it is likely that the consultant would be best equipped to deal with this scenario.

Scenario 19

Question 1: D. Not important at all

This won't achieve much. In fact, it will teach the boy to fight violence with violence. The boy should be encouraged to show he is better than them by not reacting to them. However, he should not be discouraged from protecting himself if the bullies can't see reason and attack him.

Question 2: D. Not important at all

By antagonising the bullies you have in essence become a bully yourself – solving violence with violence. Often when bullies are hurt, they take it out on people smaller than them, so this action should not be advised as it is likely to only worsen the problem.

Question 3: B. Important

The boy needs to have his confidence restored and this action may help him feel better about himself. However, you cannot be 100% certain that the bullies will not return and may find other ways to get back at the boy (e.g. cyberbullying).

Scenario 20

Question 1: B. Appropriate, but not ideal

While the end intention to hand the wallet to the police is good, it is also somewhat inappropriate to keep the wallet on you for a prolonged period of time without contacting anyone. Also, if, for instance, there was a stop and search at the concert it is possible you could be found with what appears to be stolen goods with you. Thus, it is advisable to act quicker in this situation but this needs to be balanced with your time constraints.

Question 2: D. A very inappropriate thing to do

This is very inappropriate as it avoids your responsibilities as a good citizen as well as showing a lack of integrity. While the concert may be important you still have a duty to act in a situation like this.

Question 3: C. Inappropriate, but not awful

While this will likely ensure the wallet gets to the police station as quickly as possible, this response involves handing on the responsibility to someone else rather than taking accountability yourself. Also, while it may be a good friend you cannot be entirely sure what he/she may do, thus this response still has some uncertainty attached.

Index